To Bed or Not to Bed

When I am cold
You share your heat.
When I am down
You bring me up.
I look to you when afraid,
You encourage me.
I look to you for fun
And you enjoy me.
When things are dark
You enlighten the world.
When things are dull
You entertain.
When I am out
You let me enter.
I love your love!
I love you.

Other titles in the Positively Sexual series

Extended Massive Orgasm *by* Steve Bodansky, Ph.D., and Vera Bodansky, Ph.D.
Female Ejaculation and the G-Spot *by* Deborah Sundahl
The Hot Guide to Safer Sex *by* Yvonne Fulbright, M.S. Ed.
The Illustrated Guide to Extended Massive Orgasm *by* Steve Bodansky, Ph.D., and Vera Bodansky, Ph.D.
Making Lover Better Than Ever *by* Barbara Keesling, Ph.D.
Rx Sex *by* Barbara Keesling, Ph.D.
Sensual Sex *by* Beverly Engel, MFCC
Sex Tips & Tales from Women Who Dare *edited by* Jo-Anne Baker
Sexual Healing *by* Barbara Keesling, Ph.D.
Sexual Pleasure *by* Barbara Keesling, Ph.D.
Simultaneous Orgasm *by* Michael Riskin, Ph.D., and Anita Banker-Riskin, M.A.
Tantric Sex for Women *by* Christa Schulte
Women's Sexual Passages *by* Elisabeth Davis

Ordering

Trade bookstores in the U.S. and Canada please contact:

Publishers Group West
1700 Fourth Street, Berkeley CA 94710
Phone: (800) 788-3123   Fax: (510) 528-3444

Hunter House books are available at bulk discounts for textbook course adoptions; to qualifying community, health-care, and government organizations; and for special promotions and fund-raising. For details please contact:

Special Sales Department
Hunter House Inc., PO Box 2914, Alameda CA 94501-0914
Phone: (510) 865-5282   Fax: (510) 865-4295
E-mail: ordering@hunterhouse.com

Individuals can order our books from most bookstores, by calling **(800) 266-5592**, or from our website at **www.hunterhouse.com**

TO BED OR NOT TO BED

What Men Want,
What Women Want,
How Great Sex Happens

Vera Bodansky, Ph.D.,

&

Steve Bodansky, Ph.D.

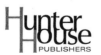

>   Hunter House Inc., Publishers
>   PO Box 2914
>   Alameda CA 94501-0914

Library of Congress Cataloging-in-Publication Data

Bodansky, Vera.
>   To bed or not to bed : what men want, what women want, how great sex happens
>   / Vera Bodansky and Steve Bodansky.— 1st ed.
>   p. cm. — (Positively sexual)
>   Includes bibliographical references and index.
>   ISBN-13: 978-0-89793-461-9 (pbk.)
>   ISBN-10: 0-89793-461-X (pbk.)
>   1. Sex. 2. Sex instruction. I. Bodansky, Steve. II. Title. III. Series.
HQ31.B59335 2006
613.9'6—dc22   2005027990

Project Credits

Cover Design:	Acquisitions Editor: Jeanne Brondino
Brian Dittmar Graphic Design	Editor: Alexandra Mummery
Book Production:	Publicist: Jillian Steinberger
Stefanie Gold and Hunter House	Customer Service Manager:
Developmental and Copy Editor:	Christina Sverdrup
Kelley Blewster	Order Fulfillment: Washul Lakdhon
Proofreader: John David Marion	Administrator: Theresa Nelson
Indexer: Nancy D. Peterson	Computer Support: Peter Eichelberger

Publisher: Kiran S. Rana

Printed and Bound by Bang Printing, Brainerd, Minnesota

Manufactured in the United States of America

9 8 7 6 5 4 3 2 1   First Edition   06 07 08 09 10

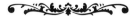

Contents

Chapter 4

Chapter 5

ᏋᎧ CONTACT INFORMATION

*If you would like information on the authors' courses, please
visit their website at* WWW.EXTENDEDMASSIVEORGASM.COM
or e-mail them at VERASTEVE@AOL.COM.

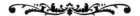

Acknowledgments

This is really more a book about love than about sex, although it is nice to have both. We would like to thank all of the people that we have used as examples in this book for their willingness to love and be loved. We are forever grateful for our education at Morehouse where we learned about how best to use the differences and similarities between men and women to make a wonderful relationship. Special thanks to Vic and Cindy Baranco for their love and guidance in the past. We are thrilled with our ongoing relationship with Regena Thomahauer, and for her continuing use of our talents. We are especially grateful to Kelly Blewster, who edited this book with such clarity and thoughtfulness. We further wish to appreciate all those lovers out there who continue to inspire us with their great examples.

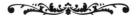

DEDICATION

to lovers everywhere

∽ Important Note ∽

The material in this book is intended to provide a review of information regarding sexuality and relationships. Every effort has been made to provide accurate and dependable information. The contents of this book have been compiled through professional research and in consultation with medical professionals. We believe that the sensuality advice given in this book poses no risk to any healthy person. However, if you have any genital infections, such as herpes, we recommend that you consult your doctor before using this book.

The publisher, authors, and editors, as well as the professionals quoted in the book, cannot be held responsible for any error, omission, professional disagreement, outdated material, or adverse outcomes that result from applying any of the information in this book. If you have questions concerning the application of the information contained in this book, consult a qualified professional.

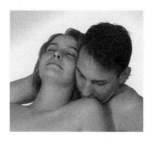

Introduction

*J*ust as in Hamlet's famous soliloquy, "To be—or not to be," the question "to bed or not to bed" could signify a life-or-death situation too. It appears that our species is producing an adequate number of offspring to put that worry to rest, but if the question is interpreted as wondering how to create real pleasure with another human being, then it takes on more importance.

The bed in the title of this book is not the literal bed—that piece of furniture most of us take for granted—just as to sleep with someone does not usually mean going unconscious (although that does happen on occasion). The bed we refer to is a metaphor for pleasure with another human being. To go to bed, as we use the phrase, means to have a sensual experience with someone, whether it is between the sheets or in the woods. (We would, however, like to point out that beds themselves can make a difference in one's sensual life. Many of us will spend thousands of dollars on a car that we use only occasionally, yet we will compromise on the quality and comfort of our bed, even though most of us will spend over a third of our lives there. A good bed with nice bedding and lots of pillows can make one's life significantly more agreeable and more pleasurable.) The chapter titles in this book all have something to do with the bed, not only because we thought the titles were appropriate and cute, but also because our expertise lies in the area of having more fun in bed. We have made a career of using the bed as a workplace where we teach others about expanding their sexual potential. Plus, our bed has been there for us whenever we have desired pleasure. We have a California-king-size bed— and in beds size does matter.

Most human beings are looking for that special someone with whom they can have a loving relationship, yet most people whom we've met have great difficulty either finding the right person or creating more intimacy in the relationship they have formed. _To Bed or Not to Bed_ tackles both of these issues, as we believe that being able to start a relationship right and being able to keep it fresh and fun are interrelated.

This book has been a collaboration between me (Steve) and my wife (Vera). We have discussed everything that has gone into print here in the same way that we discuss all matters in our lives, large or small. That is, we approach conflicts and experiences with two heads thinking together, sometimes in agreement and sometimes arguing our points until we reach some kind of mutual decision. Therefore, although it is I (Steve) who is typing and whose prose you are reading, the book is very much a team effort.

Vera and I have been married for over twenty-two years, and our relationship is better now than ever. It continues to get even better—with more intimacy, improved communication, and enhanced sex—as a result of our ongoing discussions and actions. We are not therapists or "marriage counselors," but we have been involved with thousands of students during our careers as pleasure facilitators and investigators. We both have doctorates in sensuality, and we have been involved in helping couples create more loving, healthy relationships. Our goal is to enhance couples' levels of intimacy and pleasure. Through our training and our many years of experience, we have noticed that a good relationship and pleasure go hand in hand; that is, without shared, special pleasures the relationship will suffer, and vice versa.

After we wrote two books on orgasm _(Extended Massive Orgasm_ and _The Illustrated Guide to Extended Massive Orgasm)_, we felt compelled to write a book about the possibilities of a magnificent relationship in order to complement our work and to reach more people. The result is the book you hold in your hands. This book is for anyone who wishes to enhance the intimacy, pleasure, and goodwill between two partners.

A foundational premise of this book is our belief that women are not equal to men (which also means that men are not equal to women). Everyone is not created equal, despite what Thomas Jefferson wrote in our Declaration of Independence, although being treated equally under the law is a positive political development. Men and women are different (though they are from the same planet), yet many people of both sexes have a similar goal: finding someone to be intimate with. When you are able to use the differences between the sexes to each partner's advantage, you may have a chance to actually attain your goal. As long as you are concerned about being equal and doing equal, you will be angry every time you come up against some inequality, and this will lead you away from intimacy—and away from fun, for that matter.

It is difficult to determine the causes for the differences between the sexes. An ongoing debate centers around whether the differences are caused by nature or nurture. Whether girls are born liking dolls and boys preferring toy guns and toy trucks, or whether our cultures push us in those directions. It's a challenging question to answer. Whatever the cause, the result is that girls like dolls more than boys do and boys like toy weapons more than girls do. For the purposes of this book, we are interested only in the visible effects, the results, not in their root causes. Furthermore, we are writing in generalities. Another generality, by the way, is that men are taller than women, though taken case by case, obviously, some women are taller than some men.

Although men and women are different, we do not see them dualistically—that is, as strict opposites of one another. They are actually more similar than they are dissimilar. There is no one kind of man, just as there is no one kind of woman. People come in all varieties, shapes, and sizes, and they range from extremely masculine to extremely feminine and anywhere in between. As Carol Tavris observes in *The Mismeasure of Women: Why Women Are Not the Better Sex, the Inferior Sex, or the Opposite Sex*, the male or masculine way is considered normal, making the female or feminine way different from what is considered normal. If it is different from normal then it is, in other words, abnormal. Ms. Tavris asserts, and we agree, that men are not better than women, and masculine characteristics are not better than feminine ones. She also stresses that the feminine way is not better than the masculine way. To think that women are better than men is just another way of making the male way the norm. Women have been considered the second-best sex throughout much of written history. If one sex is second-best and there are only two, that of course makes women the "worse" sex. For a long time, then, women have been considered both abnormal and worse than men. According to Leonard Schlain, author of *The Alphabet Versus the Goddess,* it has been this way since the development of the written word; others say it was the invention of the plow that doomed women. Only in recent history have the oppression and second-class treatment of women begun to be replaced with better attitudes and, thus, better circumstances.

We have done our best to write this book with as much open-mindedness as possible. No doubt it will include some sexist viewpoints that have yet to be replaced with better ones. We have concentrated mostly on the differences between the sexes that can be used for either creating fun or creating disdain. Obviously, most men relate differently to other men than they do to women, and the same goes for women. When women and men come together, we can't deny the presence of that indescribable "something"—that *vive la différence*—that can be used for pleasure or for pain. Every time a person comes into contact with someone of the other sex, even one's own children or parents, at least an undertone is present of something—an awareness—that is different from what is there when one relates to a person of the same sex. Our society has not progressed (if it is progression) to the point where we fail to notice the sex of the person with whom we are associating. There may not be sexual feelings present in all of these interactions, but feelings are there nonetheless. Life would be boring if we were all alike. Thanks to our dissimilarities, we have opportunities for exploration, excitement, wonderment, and awe. Small differences have developed into the chance to play a very big game. It takes both sexes to engage in this "woman and man" game, but one does not have to be in a relationship to play it.

One big difference between men and women is in their readiness to go to bed (though whether this has much to do with real, sustainable pleasure is debatable). Men—at least heterosexual, single, and even many married men—will almost always say yes to almost any kind of offer from almost any kind of woman, while most women are way choosier and will say yes only under the right circumstances. Unless the woman is so horny that she has lost her ability to discriminate, she is going to find the choicest mate available when she wants some, and he will have to prove his love and devotion, or at least his ability to be fun. This seems to be the case for married couples as well as first-timers. A woman has the ability to wink and say come here and make the man move toward her. A man has to work harder for sex. He often has to seduce and sweet-talk the woman into coming toward him. And so, to state it bluntly, *To Bed or Not to Bed* is at least partly about what it takes to get a woman to say yes to bed. Women really want to say yes to pleasure, but society labels a woman who says yes easily wanton or a slut or any number of other derogatory things. Therefore, men have to learn how to overcome a woman's resistances (both natural and cultural) and to develop the art of seduction.

In this book we have included information from a number of different sources, but mostly from our own experiences and those of people we know. When we have incorporated ideas from other books or teachers, we have usually cited them. The information is mostly descriptive. It is framed in terms of how we view the world, and what seems to work and not to work when men and women interact. We have tried to make it as current as possible. Each chapter contains exercises that can help you apply the book's principles to your life and relationships. When it felt appropriate to do so, we have used a slang word instead of the formal one to add special emphasis and meaning. The first chapter, "Finding and Choosing the Right Bed and Partner," is about making a space in your life for another person with whom to create the potential for a relationship and pleasure. Believe it or not, you have to make room in your life for a bed (that is, for pleasure). This chapter deals with finding a partner, and it describes some of the differences between how men and women go about achieving this goal.

Chapter 2, "Pillow Talk Plus: Tips on Communication," describes how men can become better seducers and sweet-talkers. It provides information about some of the differences between the ways women and men communicate, how to talk to and understand members of the other sex, and the games people play. Topics addressed include noticing, being a good listener, and admitting when it hurts. We also provide some examples of what not to say.

The third chapter, "Who Makes the Bed? Roles and Responsibilities in a Relationship," discusses sharing certain responsibilities that are necessary to creating a successful intimate partnership, including giving without keeping score, loving oneself as the foundation for a good relationship, taking your partner's side when he or she has a disagreement with someone else, and dealing with conflicts. It also touches on men's and women's separate roles, including in managing the emotional climate of the relationship. It deals with women's desires and how a man can help a woman fulfill those desires, thereby becoming her hero. Last but not least, it introduces the basics of good sex, including the one thing people need to know about how to reliably produce an orgasm in a woman.

Chapter 4, "Getting Ready for Bed: Overcoming Resistance to Pleasure," and Chapter 5, "Going to Bed: Sensuality and Integrity for Sexual Pleasure," take us closer to the topic of pleasure. Chapter 4 describes the various forms of resistance to pleasure and how to overcome them. An important topic is what to do about anger, the enemy of pleasure. We also present some seductive techniques specifically aimed at getting yourself ready for bed. Chapter 5, "Going to Bed: Sensuality and Integrity for Sexual Pleasure," covers a lot of sensual information, from having fun in all kinds of exotic situations, to the importance of integrity in bed, to deliberate versus default pleasure, to the use of fantasy in bed. Finally, it presents the core of our sensual teachings: how we (re)define orgasm.

Chapter 6, "Her Side of the Bed: News for Women on Achieving (and Giving) Pleasure," speaks primarily to women. It discusses how to make the best use of a woman's turn-on, why men lie to women, and how a woman can train her partner in and out of bed. It also suggests some ways for creating more fun in bed. Chapter 7, "His Side of the Bed: News for Men on Giving (and Achieving) Pleasure," is addressed primarily to men and discusses the vital importance of learning about the clitoris if a man wants to be a wonderful lover. This chapter also discusses how a man can use his penis as a sort of lie detector to help him determine a woman's true desires in bed. Although these two chapters are addressed to women and men respectively, we believe that members of each sex can learn a few new things by reading the chapter addressed to the other sex.

Chapter 8, "Under the Covers: All You Both Need to Know for Great Sex," is filled with information about how to create a better sex life. It describes what it means to be a pleasure victim and the risks and benefits of playing that role. It explains the importance of knowing and enjoying what you are doing in bed, of having confidence and integrity, of remaining playful and curious, and of focusing both your attention and your intention. Finally, it includes detailed information about how to touch a woman with an oversensitive clitoris.

There is a lot of useful sexual information scattered throughout this book. Reading it can give you a clearer idea of how to create more sensual pleasure for yourself and your partner. If you are truly interested in developing your skills as a lover and as a receiver of pleasure, we recommend the two books we wrote expressly for those purposes: *Extended Massive Orgasm* and *The Illustrated Guide to Extended Massive Orgasm*. Reading these books and this one can help you become a better lover and create a better partnership, but to reach great heights as a lover and a partner you must do the necessary work. You must practice the techniques and ideas presented in these books over time.

Not everything contained in this book will work for everyone all of the time. We have included information that has worked extremely well for us and for many other folks. We believe that almost everyone will be able to find ideas in this book that, when applied, will add more fun and more love to their lives. Although the book is written primarily for a heterosexual audience, we know a number of gay and lesbian students who could apply much of the information about the man/woman game to their lives. Since, for example, we emphasize manual stimulation of the genitals as the most efficient and competent way to create an orgasm, the information in this book and our earlier books can be useful to both gay and straight readers.

If your relationship is good already, it can be quite a challenge to make it better. Unlike when things are bad and you are trying to get back to good, when things are already good nothing is motivating you to make any changes. However, nothing is ever static: You are either going up or going down. If you are not going up, you are sliding downhill. It takes a curious and pioneering attitude to keep going for better. Reading this book can bst your efforts to become a pioneer on the quest for a more fun and rewarding life.

CHAPTER 1

Called to your side
I salute thee
With all my strength
and might.
Called to your heart
I meet thee
With all my love and
light.

Finding and Choosing the Right Bed and Partner

_T_he bed, as we mentioned in the Introduction, is our metaphor for sensual pleasure with another human being. And what is the most important component of a bed? The mattress. The mattress is what makes a bed a bed. If you were to describe your bed as, say, a waterbed, you'd be talking about the sort of mattress it has. There are all kinds of mattresses available—those filled with air and those filled with water, a few made with foam rubber, and others with "memory foam." Some European mattresses are even filled with horsehair. Mattresses range in size from twin to full to queen to king to California king. How do you know which one to choose, and once you choose one, how do you know you've made the right decision? The answer is you've got to shop around. You test them out, take one home, and if it doesn't work for you, you exchange it for another. The same goes for finding and choosing an intimate partner: You've got to shop around until you find the right one, and if that person doesn't work, you exchange him or her for a new one. The difference is that you don't have to sleep with every potential partner, as you do with a mattress, to figure out if you want to keep him or her. This chapter offers some advice on how to attract and select an intimate partner.

Over the years a lot of men and women have asked us how to get into the game. "How can I get into a relationship with a woman?" "How do I meet a good man?" It may seem a bit strange that we are asked these questions since our first two books, about extended massive orgasm, were mostly addressed to people who were already in a fully sexual and loving relationship. It's a little like George Lucas's making the last trilogy of the _Star Wars_ movies first, and then having to go back to the beginning to show how it all started by making the "prequels."

Women are everywhere (except maybe on a few golf courses). Men are everywhere too. Why, then, do people have so much trouble finding someone of the other sex to have a relationship with? A short answer is that many people are so absorbed in their own drama that they barely have time to notice— let alone pay meaningful attention to—anyone else in their universe. In addition, many women are angry at men for not being more like them, and vice versa. So even before people have a chance to get to know each other, they have created a negative mindset/expectation about the other sex that is often self-fulfilling. This chapter aims to help you change these outcomes.

∼ Hunting and Fishing ∼

As we said in the Introduction, much of this book describes how men and women are different, and how a person can play with those differences to create more pleasure, intimacy, and fun in his or her relationships with the other sex. If you're not in an intimate partnership and you'd like to change that, it may be helpful to first understand the differences between men's and women's approaches to attracting members of the other sex. This is the topic of this section. Even if you *are* in an intimate relationship, the "attraction" game is still (hopefully) a vital part of the dynamics between you and your partner, so understanding more about how both sexes play it can be useful.

Men have always assumed that they were the sex better suited to being the hunter. This may have been true for hunting woolly mammoths but does not translate as well into the hunt for a relationship. Instead, we think the woman is analogous to a fisherperson. *(Fisherman* is what most people would have said in the past, but we are trying to be politically correct and to avoid sexist language as much as possible.) The man is analogous to a fish that is hunting for worms. When he (the fish) finally finds his prey (the worm), it turns out that he has been caught by our fisherperson. We are not saying here that courtship is a predatory act, but rather we are using the analogy to illustrate the different roles the participants play. The goal on both sides is union and pleasure, which is hopefully beneficial to both parties.

Women are good at concealing both their natural ability to be the huntress/fisherperson and their voracious appetites (which we will discuss in a later chapter). The better they can wiggle that worm around while concealing the hook, the better they are at catching whatever they're looking for. The question, then, is *what are women looking for,* and *how does a man become that desired object and demonstrate that he has done so?*

Women and men, though different from each other, are first of all both human beings. All human beings (except for some psychological cases) want to be appreciated, want to be liked, and want to be loved and to love. Based on our studies, experiences, and observations, women appear to have a greater capacity than men to be cherished, adored, and found beautiful and wonderful. Women love to receive attention and to have their desires fulfilled. Shouldn't it be easy, then, just to find out what a woman wants, help her get it, and live life happily ever after? In fact, it often doesn't work that simply. Even though women crave attention and fulfillment, a lot of them don't readily give up information about *how* a man can satisfy those desires. Remember, they are the ones doing the fishing, and they are not going to show a man that shiny, sharp hook until they are sure he is the right prey.

A woman will usually give multiple tests to any man who approaches her and wants to take her bait. This means that the man who gets close enough for her to notice will somehow have to demonstrate his worth and desirability. Doing so may involve simply asking for her phone number, or it may involve having to slay fearsome dragons. A woman will usually not come right out and show her desires. She will usually not just hand a man her business card with her phone number on it and tell him the best times to call. She has made the first move by being attractive enough to draw him to her, and now he must make the next move by doing something that shows he is interested in pursuing her. As Marlene Zuk so cleverly states in her book *Sexual Selections:*

> Courtship may in fact superficially resemble predation, because one party often advances while the other party retreats. I suppose one could say that because a conflict of interest occurs between the sexes, the similarity is even greater, since obviously the hunted and hunter disagree about the best fate for the prey. But it is false to conclude that therefore females say no when they mean yes and males have to exert their will for it all to work out appropriately. The first problem is that females may be evaluating males during courtship to ensure that their mate is a good one. This may necessitate watching as he performs elaborate courtship dances and other behaviors; the male is expected to try and cut these short and attempt to mate, because he has nothing to lose and everything to gain by doing so, but the female is equally expected to make him wait until information is complete, perhaps by refusing to allow him to shortchange her. This is conflict, but it is not a miniature version of predation. It is no more indicative of the pursuer being dominant to the pursuee than a job candidate strutting his or her abilities before the boss should be.

As the old adage states, "it is the female who is chased by the male until she catches him."

Not every woman, of course, is going to follow these covert tactics in every situation. Sometimes a woman sees someone she likes and wants and is more overt in her approach. The rules a woman plays by in the game of love depend on so many factors—her age, the peer pressure on her, the culture she belongs to—that they cannot be predicted for any specific woman or circumstance. Still, in general, the observations we make here apply. We base them on what we have noticed in many of our students and other people over many years. We also have a theory about *why* the two sexes have developed these strategies: It is because women and girls aren't included in "the club." Until recently, if things have changed at all, more new parents have said, "It's a boy!" more proudly than "It's a girl!" For the past several thousand years human males have been born into a world where they were the "right" sex. Boys had no reason to doubt this assumption; why should they? If someone tells you from the get-go that you are the best and are part of the club, it must be true. Girls, with good reason, have often felt wronged by being the number-two sex. (Girl babies are still often killed in China, where parents can have only one child, and in India.) Because girls and women have not been members of the club, they have often had to resort to behind-the-scenes maneuvering to get their needs and desires met. Of course, not every man is aboveboard and not every woman is sneaky, but we have noticed that, especially in how the two genders relate to each other, these behaviors are quite evident and par for the course. We will spend more time describing why men lie when in relationships in Chapter 6, "Her Side of the Bed."

∼ White-Knight Syndrome ∼

Men often flunk the tests women give them without even realizing they were being tested. They end up wondering why they were dumped. Testing a man and then breaking it off with him when he fails may be a useful technique for weeding out poor choices, but often a woman will dump a man for some little thing he did or did not do, or for some minor lack of judgment. We have a friend who will dump a man for the slightest bad habit. She was in love with a man until, on one of their first trips together, he flossed his teeth in bed.

Instead of either changing her viewpoint and deciding that this was a healthy and actually cute habit, or training him to change his behavior (we talk more about training later), she decided his behavior was disgusting and broke things off with him. She never even told him why she didn't want to see him again. If a woman (or a man, for that matter) is going to dump somebody, it is the friendly thing to do to let him know what he did wrong, so that maybe the next time, with the next woman, he will avoid the same mistake.

Another time, when our friend was in love, her then-boyfriend phoned and said he had some presents for her. When he arrived at her house, he gave her one rose. Instead of being thankful that he brought her a flower, she was pissed that he said "presents" (plural) and then showed up with only one. She could have told him right away that the flower was beautiful and she really appreciated it—and also that she felt he could have communicated better. She might have kindly told him that instead of saying "presents" he could have said he had "something" for her, and that receiving the flower would have been even more fun for her with that setup. She did not completely break up with him for this transgression, but he was definitely on the way out.

We call this behavior the white-knight syndrome—that is, finding each potential relationship wrong for a different reason every time. It's as though the woman is looking for a perfect man, her prince or knight in shining armor. In fact, such a man does not exist; there are only frogs out there, and a woman has to make her white knight out of one of them.

Rather than dumping a guy for making a minor transgression, especially if he shows some potential, another choice may be to decide to make a mensch out of him. *(Mensch* is a Yiddish word for an all-around decent human being.) A woman does this by telling the man how he is doing well and by showing him how he can improve his game when he makes a mistake. This is called training, and all men need it. If you are a woman and want a great man, it is up to you to train him for yourself. (We include some proven techniques for training and communicating with your partner in the chapters "Her Side of the Bed" and "Under the Covers.") You have probably heard women say that "all the good men are taken." Every "good man" is that way because some woman decided to take him on and give him enough loving attention to transform him into what she wanted him to be. This is what we mean by "training."

All single guys are frogs—some with more warts and bad habits than others—but they are all trainable to some extent. Even if a woman gets a man who has been trained by another woman, the new woman is still going to have to put some work into him to get him to be the right man for her.

Justin Sterling writes in his book *What Really Works with Men* that men are not very trainable; whatever state you find him in, do not expect him to change. He says a man will not grow into a prince, but if you find one whose viewpoints are compatible with yours, you can live a happy life together. This is good information. It is true that to expect to change a man into a completely different person is wishful thinking. However, we believe that men are somewhat more trainable than Mr. Sterling says. We believe that a good woman can have a huge impact in making a mensch out of her man. Regena Thomashauer writes in *Mama Gena's Owner's and Operator's Guide to Men* that to believe in the Sleeping Beauty myth and wait for Prince Charming to come around and wake you up is setting yourself up for failure. She says that to some extent a woman has to know what she wants and then go out into the world and find it or create it by using her abilities to attract and to have pleasure. In our view, most men's actual trainability probably lies somewhere between the total makeover that Ms. Thomashauer suggests is possible and the "nontrainability" that Mr. Sterling believes is the reality. We believe that a woman can find a man who is willing to go along on her ride—or at least a man whose ride is compatible with hers—and fine-tune him to be a prince.

It is also true that a number of men out there are looking for that "perfect" woman. However, many of these men can easily be had. When a woman finds herself to be "perfect" the way she is—when finds herself attractive and she actually likes herself and the way she looks and acts—she will attract men who feel the same way about her. Of course, the occasional man exists who habitually finds his partner lacking in some area and thus quickly moves on, but we have noticed that this behavior is a lot more rare in men than in women.

When a person is fishing, they don't keep every fish they catch. Sometimes the fish is too big, and other times the fish is just not the type they wanted. Sometimes the fish is too small. (No pun intended, we're just talking about fish here. Most men with small penises feel hexed by that fact, but the truth is, once a man learns how to pleasure a woman's clitoris, and a woman learns how to push out and collapse her vaginal walls, she will not care about the size of his organ. We describe these techniques in Chapters 6 and 7.) When this happens the fisherperson throws the fish back into the sea, puts some new bait on the hook, and fishes some more. If a man keeps finding himself being thrown back into the sea, he would be wise to learn if there's a recurring theme in his breakups and to do what it takes to become a better catch. If he wants to improve his game it would be wise for him to ask the woman what he could have done better or where he failed with her. But if he does not want to go directly to the woman who has just rejected him, he can use other resources, such as female relatives or wives of friends, to help him boost his game. He should get help wherever he can.

∾ The Eye of the Beholder ∾

Men, it's a fact: How you present yourself matters. It's important to understand that most women like to dress up from time to time, and when they do they don't want the man they are with to look unkempt. He actually becomes a part of her look. She sees him as other women do: as a reflection of her appearance. Many women have enjoyed dressing up ever since they changed outfits on their dolls as little girls. When women get married they may spend thousands of dollars on a wedding dress that will be worn only once. Most men think this is absolutely crazy, yet women won't think twice about it. Since childhood they have nursed the fantasy of their special white wedding dress, and when the time is right they don't want to miss the opportunity.

If grooming and dressing aren't your strong suits, maybe you have a sister who can advise you. Perhaps one of your married friend's wives will help you out, maybe even take you shopping. When Vera and I take walks we often notice guys who are obviously single; they are dressed in such a way that you just know they don't have a woman paying attention to them. Vera says they look like unmade beds (a suitable metaphor for this book). Not every well-dressed man you see is in a relationship with a woman—certainly lots of gay men know how to dress—but it does seem that many heterosexual men are missing the gene for how to dress and make the most of their appearance.

When Vera found me, I didn't have much of a wardrobe. I didn't own a suit or even a sport jacket. I had numerous white gym socks with different-colored bands at the top, and I often wore mismatched pairs of these. In the ten years prior to meeting Vera I had been married and had lived with two women, yet I was still quite froggy. Although I did not have money or a regular job, I was in good physical shape and well educated, but I still looked like one of those unmade beds. Luckily for me, Vera was able to see past the clothing and the lack of funds to realize that I had some raw potential that she could help bring out. I was living communally, so there were many women available for me to have fun with, but Vera took more interest in me than any of the other women did. She gradually helped me change my appearance so that I dressed better, wore matching socks, and finally began looking like a made bed. (It took her a number of years, however, to get me to buy and wear a suit.)

Most women can tell when a guy is single and has never been in a serious relationship just by the way he is dressed and how he looks. It's just human nature, but women tend to avoid such a man. They feel that if no one else has found him appealing, there must be a good reason why. It is like the empty-restaurant scenario. If you are in a city or town that you have never visited before and are looking for a place to eat, would you pick a restaurant that was empty or one that was nearly full of customers? The answer is obvious. Similarly, women can smell the "scent of pussy" on a man. Men who are or have been with other women become more desirable to them. This is important for guys to understand. A lot of men want to go out with only the prettiest, most popular women, and since these types are usually taken or are unreachable, such men may choose not to date at all. This is a mistake. If a man goes out with any woman, even one who may not be stunningly beautiful, it makes him much more desirable to other women. Also, he may be surprised and may learn to be less shallow; he may discover that beauty is only skin-deep and that he can have a great time with many different kinds of women. It is also true that the more positive attention people get, the more attractive they become. Besides, drop-dead beautiful women can often be stuck-up, narcissistic, and not much fun. To keep going after this type of woman may be more painful than it is pleasurable.

When a woman keeps finding herself with men who don't call her back after or even before a first date, or who turn out to be bad choices, she might begin to wonder what she can do differently to raise the standard of her catch.

We have found that we usually attract people according to how we feel about ourselves. Women often attract lousy choices because they feel lousy about themselves. They do not like themselves very much, and as a result attract men who do not like them very much either. If this happens it is time to regroup and begin to explore loving oneself more. Two of the exercises we've included at the end of this chapter, "Setting the Space for Pleasure" and "Visual Investigation," are particularly good for helping people who are learning to love themselves more. Designed for both men and women, they will continue to improve one's self-image the more one performs them.

People have many characteristics that are fixable. They also have traits that are either unfixable or are such an essential part of themselves that to attempt to change them would be counterproductive. Things like bad breath or a dorky haircut or outdated clothes are easily altered. Other qualities, like acting macho, failing to be a good listener, or being overly sexist, are more difficult to change, but trying to do so may definitely be beneficial to the goal. However, if you love music and dislike sports, for example, we do not recommend trying to change those qualities just because the women or men you have been attracted to so far don't share your passions. It's better to go to a different sea or pond instead of the same sports bar you've been going to, and to look for different types of people to date. We have a male friend who thought a woman he was dating should not wear high-heeled shoes or so much makeup. When it is still early in a potential relationship we believe it is wise to refrain from communicating your negative prejudices about the other person until you know each other better. After more than twenty years of marriage to Vera, at times I may prefer that she wear less makeup or wear more comfortable shoes, but she will usually let me know it is none of my business. Most women do not seem to appreciate it when men enter this realm, while most men who live with a woman will let her influence how he dresses and how he looks. Women will more often turn to other women or sometimes to a gay man than they will to their own partners for advice on grooming and appearance.

～ Some Rules of the Game ～

Once a man has dealt with basics like grooming and appearance, what should he do in a social setting when he spots an attractive woman he'd like to meet?

The "rules" we outline here are not written in stone, of course, but they tend to apply in most circumstances and for most people. In most cases, a man has to make the overture in order for a woman to feel safe to play and to show more appetite. At a dance it is usually expected that the man approach the woman and ask her to dance. If two people meet at a bar, the man is expected to offer to buy her a drink or to start a conversation. If a guy, no matter how cute how he is, just sits there, it is highly unlikely that any woman will approach him and start to flirt unless he happens to be a famous actor or athlete. So although we have said that women are ultimately the hunters, what this means is they are wiggling their bait to initiate contact or attract attention. It is still the man's job to look for potential bait, meaning he has to keep his eyes and ears open to be a good fish.

Women look for all kinds of relationships. The stereotype is that women look for a lifetime mate while men are just looking for some place to plant their seed. That is not always the case. Different women are looking for different types of relationships, ranging from marriage to a one-night fling. The same is true of men; some just want a casual affair and others want the whole wonderful relationship thing. If a man uses his wits and really tunes in to the woman he is interacting with, he can decipher which type of relationship she's looking for and can act accordingly. The same is true for women. This book primarily targets readers who are interested in more than a shallow, one-time fling (although there is nothing wrong with that style of relating). In reality, we doubt that most people who want only a taste would even have picked up a book about how to make and maintain a great relationship.

∾ Turn-On: A Woman's Natural Talent ∾

A powerful and turned-on woman entrances men, and as a result they will respond to her goals and desires. A woman is turned on when she is in agreement with her desires, when she likes herself, and when she is able to send a signal or stimulate a response in another person (male or female), either sexually or otherwise. By "in agreement with" we mean she finds her desires, whether physical, intellectual, creative, or emotional, to be coming from a place that is truthful to who she is. She does not regard herself as "unnatural"; rather, she likes how she feels and what she wants. She is in harmony with her wants, goals, and appetites. For example, a woman may crave lobster, but if she finds this desire inappropriate because lobster is expensive, and if she denies herself because she thinks that her ordering it will scare the man away by revealing her appetites, she will not come across as turned on. On the other hand, if she exposes her appetite by pleasurably ordering what she really wants, she will be demonstrating turn-on, and her date will enjoy fulfilling her desires. This is just an example. A woman who wants a hamburger or a salad can order it and be turned on; it just depends on what she wants and whether she is willing to ask for it.

Sexually speaking, all female mammals go into estrus, or heat, a state in which the body is able to stimulate a male of the same species to sexual excitement either through the release of pheromones, through scent, visually, or otherwise. Estrus occurs in most species in a monthly or yearly cycle. Male mammals do not have this ability; they can only respond to female heat. According to Helen Fisher, in her book *The Sex Contract,* female humans have the additional ability to create volitional heat; that is, they can cause this excitement at any time of the month or year. Combined with their beingness (a state you might think of as being comfortable with oneself) and with their ability to show appreciation to men, women can use this turn-on to cause men (and even other women) to respond to their desires and goals with positive action.

Another important premise of this book is that men find a great sense of purpose—maybe even their *greatest* sense of purpose—in fulfilling women's desires and goals. We delve deeper into this topic in Chapter 2, but for now let us just say that, based on our observations, the relationships that last longest and are most successful are those in which the woman is getting her goals fulfilled and the man is helping her in that quest. This does not mean that men don't have meaningful desires of their own or that men have to be in relationships to live productive lives. In a successful relationship both parties get their goals and wants fulfilled, and we have found that a great place to start is in meeting the woman's.

Doubt and anger are turn-on's biggest enemies. A woman who doubts her turn-on and her attractiveness sends mixed signals and consequently will have difficulty getting her man to do her bidding. And even if a woman's anger is covert, a man will still be prevented from picking up on her turn-on and will probably respond with either anger of his own or perhaps just with apathy. Anger coming from either party in a relationship is a major barrier to a great union. We explore anger in more detail in Chapter 4.

We have known many guys who said they were never going to get married and a few weeks later turned up engaged. This phenomenon is a powerful testimony to the power of a woman's turn-on. I remember saying when I was twenty years old and "green" that I would never get married. A few months later I was engaged—after making the proper proposal, complete with ring—and totally enthralled with the idea of marriage and everything that went with it. Women can take heart at this ability of theirs to sway a man. I have a cousin who was a confirmed bachelor. Then in his forties he met a woman who knew right away that he was the man for her, even though he was sexist and stand-offish. She explained to her mother how she felt about him, even though he seemed so resistant to the idea of a relationship. Her mother told her not to worry, that men do not know what they want, and it was up to her to show him. The daughter did what her mother suggested, staying friendly, kind, and loving and not getting upset over his resistances. Soon they were engaged, got married, had two kids, and were living very rich and gratifying lives. He was a renowned scientist and she worked for the United Nations. Together they take skiing vacations, go to the opera, travel abroad, and share many common interests that they would have missed out on if she had given up easily. They have been happily married for over thirty years.

∽ The Importance of Enthusiasm ∽

A lot of women are looking for men who appear "alive" and who will be of some use to them, whether that means showing them a fun time today or romancing them in the future. The best thing a man can do to show a woman he has something to offer is to be enthusiastic about whatever he is doing, even if it is just washing his car or walking his dog. A woman may notice his enthusiasm and perhaps wonder how she can put it to her good use. When a woman who is hunting spots an enthusiastic man, she may work her turn-on and dangle some bait—like a smile, a wink, or a glance—that a conscious man will be able to pick up on as a signal to approach her.

We asked our pretty friend Celia what she does to get a guy to notice her when she is interested in him. She told us she likes to use the direct approach. As it turns out, though, her "direct" approach is not so direct. She said she usually sits next to him and waits for him to start talking to her. After talking with him for a while, if she likes him, she will allow him to get to know her better, and if she isn't interested, she will move on to her next "catch." One time, while waiting in the lobby of a hotel, she noticed a cute guy whom she wanted to draw into her net. Acting like she didn't see him, she made a call on her cell phone. While talking, she moved closer and closer toward him until she finally bumped into him. She apologized for not seeing him, and he quickly jumped on the bait; they started talking and he soon asked if he could see her later.

If a man is unconscious of what is going on around him, he might just miss that one woman who passes him in the supermarket or stands next to him in line at the DMV and who would love to get together for a date. Most people remain unaware and unconscious by staying in their heads—that is, by thinking about their everyday problems and recycling past failures, paying only enough attention to their environment to avoid bumping into walls or poles. The perfect woman could walk right past and go unnoticed.

We have a friend in his early twenties whom we will call Howard. Howard falls in love with beautiful women every other day, on the surface at least. He goes after some of them with gusto and trepidation. He has never had a full relationship with a woman, and he worries that this will always be the case. He is not bad-looking and is a genuinely loving and caring person who will one day make a wonderful husband. The problem is that he comes on to women too strongly, and they wind up running from him either right away or soon thereafter. Furthermore, the women he falls in love with are often the most unobtainable ones, such as the beautiful opera singer or the tall, blonde, leggy model. One time he fell in love with "the most beautiful woman in all of India." He writes them poetry about his love, follows them all over the countryside, and brings them gifts, yet he is still rejected.

Vera and I are not psychologists or therapists, and we are not here to "fix" anyone. However, we have noticed that, if he wished to, Howard could become more desirable prey than he has been so far. Part of this will occur naturally as he grows older and more mature. What else can he do, though, that will make him more desirable now? First of all, he can put some of that enthusiastic attention on women who will appreciate it. There is no shortage of women who are looking for men, either to date or to be in a relationship with. Howard seems to go for the prettiest one, and soon he wants her to marry him. He can shorten his goal to that of just having fun today and then see where things go.

To meet women, Howard could take advantage of opportunities presented in his everyday life (like we pointed out above, paying attention to his surroundings when he's just going about his business), or he could seek out new places where there are plenty of available women. Many matchmaking sites now exist on the Internet where all one has to do is sign up, write a profile, and pay a few dollars to join. Blind dates may not always work out, but if a person goes on a number of them, sooner or later he or she will find a good match. My parents met on a blind date and they have been married for more than fifty-nine years. We have met many couples who originally got together on a blind date. So ask your friends to set you up, or sign up with an Internet dating service. However you do it, get out there and make a real effort to find someone.

⏤ Take Your Swings ⏤

So now that you've decided to get into the game, you have to go up to the plate and take your swings. In order to find or be found by someone, you have to get out there, take some risks, and either look for that bait or dangle a bait that will attract some bites. By taking risks, we mean you have to be willing to get rejected. A man has to get out there and make some offers to women. Women have to get out there and be attractive enough so men will make them offers, or, if they want to make an offer, they have to realize that the more attractive they feel and act the better the chance that their offer will be accepted. Let us reemphasize that by "attractive" we don't mean a woman has to look like a Hollywood movie star or a New York model; it means liking and even loving herself the way she is, whatever her physical attributes.

Being rejected, while it may not be fun, does at least indicate that you are playing the game. Like any good salesperson knows, each "no" takes you one step closer to "yes." The more offers to the more people you make, the greater are your chances of hearing yes. The law of percentages says that sooner or later someone will surprise you and accept your offer. Men, you have at least two choices to make if a woman rejects your offer. First, you can play with her about the rejection and use it in your seduction of her (a technique we explain in the next chapter). Or you can thank her for her response and move on with your search.

When taking your swings, as we illustrated with Howard and have alluded to throughout the chapter, it is also a good idea to limit your search to an appropriate place and type of person. It wouldn't make sense for a twenty-five-year-old guy to look for dates at a senior's residential home even though there are nine women to every man at most of them. Go where women are hunting, such as a matchmaking site on the Internet or a class at a local college in a field that you enjoy. Many women love to dance and appreciate any man who does, so a great place to meet women would be at a dance or a dance class.

One of our students, whom we'll call Stan, had been divorced for many years and lived alone. Besides his full-time job, as an artistic hobby he made guitars from scratch. First, he would find the right tree from which to harvest the wood; then he had to allow many months for the cut lumber to cure. He furnished his home with all kinds of specialty tools that he needed to turn the seasoned piece of lumber into a thing of beauty and elegance that produced the perfect pitch and sound. The whole process of making a single one of these masterful instruments took about a year, during which time he worked every evening. The hobby took all his time and energy, as well as all the space in his home except for bed, kitchen, and bathroom. Stan very much wanted a relationship, and his enthusiasm and attention to detail made him nearly a perfect catch. However, on the few occasions when he met women whom he wanted to get to know better, once he'd shown them his home and his guitars they were scared off because they thought there was no room in his life or home for them. Eventually Stan took up ballroom dancing. Being the enthusiastic, monomaniacal person he was, he totally gave up making guitars and went out every evening to classes and dances. He became an expert dancer and began meeting many women. He was pursued by a number of them until one pinned him down and hooked him. Time will tell whether he continues his nightly dancing career or devotes all of his attention to his new woman friend.

It doesn't matter what the hobby is; if both of you like it, then you will start a relationship with something in common, which will make for a happier union down the line. Another client of ours, Robert, had trouble meeting women, and when he did meet them he lacked enough confidence and willingness to take risks to attract their attention or to follow up on their "bait wiggling." He took a sexuality class from us, which gave him enough confidence to get out and take some chances with women (more on the connection between sexual skill and confidence appears in the next section). So he signed up for a class in making stained-glass windows. There were about twelve people in the class, ten of whom were women. He dated a couple of them and ended up finding the love of his life, whom he is still with ten years later. They are still making stained-glass windows together.

A woman who wants to find men can find them everywhere, if she is conscious. She can take a class in a subject that men are attracted to. A friend of ours took a class in welding, where she met her future husband. We know of women who go to supermarkets in expensive neighborhoods, scope out the single guys, meet one of them "accidentally on purpose," and end up dating him. Men really are almost everywhere, just as women are; one simply has to take some risks, introduce oneself, and see what happens.

∼ Confidence and Risk-Taking ∼

Because they're so important when trying to meet a potential partner, let's talk some more about confidence and risk-taking. Robert would probably have been unable to get into a great relationship if he had lacked the confidence and self-assurance he acquired by taking our private instructions on how to please a woman sexually. Men, it is of utmost importance to learn how to gratify a woman sexually and to be able to really devote your attention to her, not only in bed but also in all areas of life. This book and our other ones can help you do that.

In general, men are quite uninformed about how to please a woman sexually. When I met my first wife, at age nineteen, I knew nothing about how to give a woman pleasure. I had always liked girls, but I was very shy as a teenager. I went to an all-boys high school, and when we had dances with the girls' schools I stayed away because I was afraid of what to say and because I thought I couldn't dance very well. Talking and dancing are two skills that many girls and women place a lot of importance on. Developing confidence in all three areas (sexuality, talking, and dancing) is recommended if a man seriously wants to meet women and hit it off with them.

Once I got to college I began interacting with women more. I went to dances and thus got better at dancing because I was doing it more. I did not date a lot during my first two years, but I did go out with a few girls and had a relationship with one for a few months. As I said, I knew nothing about how to give a woman pleasure, but I wanted to go all the way with my girlfriend. She didn't want to, and, lacking knowledge about how to properly seduce a woman, I was unable to change her mind. I broke up with her. Even though I wanted to lose my virginity, ultimately I decided that having a girlfriend was more important to me. I got into agreement with my predicament and came to the decision that I would not put pressure on myself or my next girlfriend to go all the way. Almost immediately I found myself playing with a cute Scottish terrier whose owner was a pretty girl sitting on the steps of the student union (the dog, of course, was part of her bait). We talked for a while and agreed to meet at the cafeteria later that day.

The only problem (if it was a problem) with my new, aggressive approach to meeting women was that I met someone on my first attempt. We started seeing each other, fell in love, each lost our virginity, and eventually got married. Now that I had found a woman—or one had found me—I was no longer in the "looking" game. I was very glad indeed that I had a relationship. We got along well, cuddled a lot, and had fun together. Neither of us knew much about sensuality. We moved to Europe for a couple of years after college, and when we came back to the United States, the relationship went south, though we both tried. Only after we broke up did I begin my sensual education, learning how to gratify a woman and about the importance of the clitoris.

Shortly after the marriage ended I moved into a commune in Brooklyn where the residents had in common the desire to learn more about sex and sensuality. I shared a room with a young lady and had fun exploring pleasure with a number of women who lived there. This was in the early 1970s, when people were more open to sexual exploration. One afternoon I went to the library to find a book on plumbing, as we were having some plumbing problems at the house. I asked a beautiful young girl who worked at the library for some help in finding the book I needed. She never did find the book; I'm not sure if it was because we got sidetracked or because the library didn't have any plumbing books. Anyway, I asked her for her phone number, called her that evening, and we made a date to go out. We began seeing each other regularly. She was younger than I, and very quick, adventurous, and ready to play. I was about twenty-five and by then knew how to pleasure a woman.

Up to that time, I had aggressively hit on only two women, and both times it developed into a five-year relationship. The point of my story is not to say that every time you flirt and show a woman some attention it will lead to something more. Rather, my experiences taught me that if I had never asked, nothing would have happened. They also taught me to be careful of what you wish for, because you just might get it. I had lived my first nineteen years afraid of talking to girls and afraid of being rejected. I was a good-looking, intelligent, nice guy. Plenty of girls would have said yes to me; I just never asked. Once I was willing to be rejected and to go out on a limb and ask for a woman's phone number or ask to see her later, it all worked like a charm. We have a friend who flirted with women all the time. Immediately after meeting them he would ask them to go out, ask for their phone number, even ask them to marry him. He was rejected 95 percent of the time, but with those odds if he'd asked out twenty women a week, he would have had a date every week.

Once you've been hooked, the next question is whether she'll keep you or throw you back into the sea. That depends on your responses, your actions, and your level of integrity. And your responses and actions will depend in part on the woman—specifically, on her desires and goals and on how much of herself she is willing to expose. Sometimes you may feel that you've been caught by the wrong woman and wish to escape. (As we touched on above, a woman can often overcome these feelings in a man by demonstrating genuine turn-on.) It is best to use your integrity to tell her the truth without anger, to approve of and appreciate all that you like about her, and also to politely report any negative feelings and responses that come up for you. If a woman is moving too fast in terms of seeking a commitment, let her know that you like her but are not ready to move that quickly. This shows her where you stand.

It allows her to either up her ante, pass on you altogether, or continue more slowly.

Obviously, women experience rejection too, whether it takes the form of failing to attract the man they've wiggled their bait for or being dumped after one or more dates. The reasons for a man's rejection of a woman can be manifold. He may be a shallow guy who is interested only in women who look like models. He may simply feel that she and he make a bad match. It may be that he is too timid to follow up on the bait offered. Or it may be because the woman is very angry at men or has doubts about her attractiveness. If she is conscious, a woman can usually realize what kind of man she is dealing with soon after meeting him. By "conscious" we mean being aware of what is going on outside of oneself and really tuning in to the other person's behavior and not just his words. As we mentioned earlier, many people are so wrapped up in themselves and how they're coming across to the person they're with that they fail to really notice the other person. A cousin of mine fell in love with a man who was a sweet-talker. Because she refused to see him for who he really was, she lent him money repeatedly, all the while falling for his lines about how much in love he was with her. After taking most of her savings, he dumped her and disappeared. Her friends had told her to watch out for this guy, but she didn't believe them. Perhaps "love" had made her blind.

Most men are not very good at lying to women. Any woman who is sure of herself will be able to see a man for who he is. It is always a good idea to pay attention to the actions and behaviors of the person you're interacting with and to notice whether what they say is in agreement with what they do. However, if a woman is plagued with self-doubt and a lack of self-worth, she may stay with a guy even if she has figured out that he's shallow, knowing full well the probable outcome. This is where the importance of confidence for women comes in. Even a good guy will sense if a woman has low self-worth, and depending on how pervasive it is, he will be repulsed by it. Needy and clingy women have the effect of causing men to withdraw. It is low self-worth that makes a woman feel she *needs* a man. Instead of coming from a place of desire, she is coming from a place of scarcity, and that is a turn-off. A woman who likes herself and her body is attractive to others. She does not have to be a classic beauty to attract a good catch. All she has to do to keep a good man is to give him enough "wins"—primarily by being happy—and to avoid coming across as needy. The exercises we've included at the end of this chapter can help a woman feel good about herself and thus boost her sex appeal.

∽ Choosing the Right Partner ∽

Women, any relationship will work best when you choose a man who is already close to what you want in a partner. As we discussed earlier, although a woman can train a man to alter some of his behaviors, his basic personality won't change very much. You can teach a man to put the toilet seat down when he's finished in the bathroom, for example, but you won't be able to make him into something he is not. He will not become outgoing if he is an introvert, and he will not become a quiet, stay-at-home sort if he is a partier and a playboy. It is best for a woman to have some flexibility in terms of her preferences; that is, she will have greater luck finding a good match if she doesn't make her list of desired characteristics so restrictive that it would be impossible for any one man to fill. Choose your priorities wisely. It is reasonable to want a man who treats you well, is outgoing, and wants children, for example, but to specify that he be six feet two, have blue eyes, and drive a Mercedes might be too limiting.

An attractive woman whom we knew was in love with a man who didn't want to settle down with just one woman. She wanted him to stop seeing other women and to marry her. They even lived together, with her supporting him financially. However, he simply was not a one-woman guy, and her nurturing the hope and expectation that he might change caused her great pain and anguish. He told her she was a great lover as well his best friend and confidant, but he did not want her as his wife. In such a case a person would do best to move on—to kick him out of her house and find a guy who really wants her. Alternatively, she could make an effort to change her hopes and expectations and enjoy her lover for who he is, but such a scenario is more difficult and in most cases unrealistic.

Our friend's story is an illustration of a person who wasn't being choosy enough. She let herself continue to suffer because she kept wishing and hoping he'd change, rather than seeing him for who he was, deciding he and she were incompatible, and moving on. On the flip side, we have met countless women and men who were so choosy about potential mates that they virtually eliminated the whole human race from contention. They seemed to be hoping for an influx of possible dating choices from some parallel universe.

To gauge whether a relationship with a potential partner will be successful, it is good to know certain things about yourself and about the other person before you tie the knot. Yaacov and Sue Deyo have written an excellent book, _Speed Dating,_ about finding out as early as possible in the dating process whether the person would make a logical and healthy partner for you. Remember what we said about choosing your priorities? It is way more important to consider a person's character than it is to concern yourself with what kind of accessories they come with. We recommend looking for someone who has character traits that are compatible with who you are—such as being generous and responsible, if those qualities are important to you—rather than worrying about whether they're good-looking and drive a flashy car. You can tell a lot more about a person by noticing what they do and how they treat others rather than relying on what they say. This is especially true at first, since many men will say almost anything to get a woman to go to bed with them. We also recommend looking for someone whose long-term goals and life choices are compatible with yours, or at least someone whose goals and choices you can support and who will support yours. The Deyos recommend knowing before you date someone what you're looking for in a partner and ending a relationship early if the other person doesn't have the characteristics you value. Regarding sexual chemistry, they believe, as we do, that it is nice, but not something to base a lifetime relationship on.

We differ with the Deyos on one point: whether to go to bed with someone before you know for sure that he or she is the one. The Deyos recommend waiting, but we believe the choice can depend on a number of factors. When both people are sexually confident and know what they are doing in bed, we do not think it spells doom for the relationship if they choose to enjoy some sensual pleasures with each other. We agree with the Deyos that engaging in intercourse is probably not a good idea too early in a relationship, but we believe that having fun with one another and manually giving each other orgasmic pleasure can help two people decide whether or not to get more seriously involved. We do believe that if at least one of the individuals is sexually naïve, then going to bed early in the relationship might be damaging to the couple's future togetherness.

At what point, then, would going to bed be a good choice or a bad choice? This depends on the individuals involved. We have met a number of women who did not like the way certain men made love to them or even kissed them and who used that as an excuse to dump them. On the flip side, we haven't met many men who had a wonderful time in bed with a woman, even early in a relationship, and then who wound up dumping her for going to bed with him. If having sex "too early" makes a man lose interest, then he probably wasn't the right guy anyhow. A woman is best served by realizing this, moving on, and being thankful for discovering it early.

It can be a good idea to wait to get to know a person before exposing one's genitals and heart to him or her. If one truly likes a person and thinks a person could be "the one," then waiting and just enjoying his or her company without jumping into bed might be the best path. That way, two people can get to know each other fully without the charge of sexual performance influencing their decisions. This is especially true if a person is less than confident about his or her ability to pleasure and be pleasured. There also must be some physical attraction between two people, which sometimes can develop over time as they get to know and care for each other. Remember, too, that you don't have to be involved with Brad Pitt or Catherine Zeta-Jones to find the person attractive.

Through our years of teaching many people how to become better lovers, we have been pleased to observe that couples who may be discontented with their sex life can learn new skills and as a result become thrilled with each other's sexual abilities and attentions, whether they've been together for years or are just starting a new relationship. So it turns out that you *can* teach an old couple new tricks to aid them in their quest for intimacy, and you can also teach a new couple some fine techniques. Developing communication skills is especially useful for improving a couple's level of satisfaction in bed. We have included a number of exercises in later chapters for this precise purpose.

Sometimes we've had students who began their relationship as sexual research partners. They did not intend to fall in love with each other but rather had planned to work together to learn how to experience more pleasure in bed and to become better lovers. Usually this sort of arrangement lasts for a few months till one of them becomes romantically involved with another person. In several cases, however, we've seen the relationship between research partners evolve into a full, romantic love story.

~

The next chapter describes some of the different ways in which men and women communicate. It also offers some very useful techniques that can help you get closer to someone and perhaps even persuade him or her to go to bed with you. We think it is okay to seduce and "manipulate" a person for his or her pleasure and welfare. We obviously do not condone seduction and manipulation that lead to a person's doing something they later regret or that cause anyone harm.

✧ EXERCISE 1A ✧
Setting a Space for Pleasure

This exercise can be done either on its own or as a preliminary to the visual-investigation exercise (Exercise 1B) or the self-pleasure exercises (Exercises 6A and 7A).

Most people who are expecting a visitor spend a little time and energy fixing up their home. The more special and important we consider the visitor, the more attention we devote to making our home look and feel just right. The purpose of this exercise is to create a special space in your home and to do so with more loving attention than normal. Select a room. Pretend that someone very special is coming to visit and that you have thirty minutes to an hour to clean and prepare this space for the occasion. Next, gather or purchase at least one item to please each of your five senses, plus something to stimulate your imagination or conceptual thought. The items should be things that you find particularly sensual and pleasurable. For example, you might select some compelling music for your auditory sense, a beautiful item made of silk, velvet, or ivory to please your sense of touch, fresh flowers for your sense of smell, a lovely candle for your visual sense, and some fresh fruit or delicious chocolates to stimulate your sense of taste. To please your imagination you might select a romance novel, a video, or just your personal fantasies. Now spend a few minutes enjoying each item.

✧ EXERCISE 1B ✧
Visual Investigation

This is the exercise that we believe is the most beneficial to helping people learn to love themselves more. The assignment is for you to look at your body with only loving and approving eyes; you are to find everything good about it and to love each part. Use both a full-length mirror and a hand mirror so you can examine your whole body from all kinds of angles. We usually recommend undressing and doing the exercise in the nude, but it also works to do it with some clothes on. Check out places that you normally don't look at, including your genitals.

The exercise may be difficult, but chances are you can find at least one part of your body that you can approve of and like. Maybe it's your broad shoulders, or your perfectly shaped feet, or your sturdy legs that do such a good job of getting you where you need to go. Whatever it is, start there. Bit by bit you'll find each part a little easier to love, until eventually you'll be able to admit that you really like the whole package. Do the exercise often, emphasizing different areas of the body each time. Be creative and experiment in as many different ways as you can think of. Don't be discouraged if approving of your body doesn't come easily. Hang in there and keep doing the exercise; the results will be well worth the effort. It is amazing how a person's sex appeal improves when he or she has a positive self-image. Use this opportunity to learn to love yourself more.

✧ EXERCISE 1C ✧
Gratitude List

Writing a gratitude list is simple, fun, and allows us to focus on the good parts of our lives instead of on our problems and negative feelings. Start by writing "I am grateful for..." and then list whatever you truly appreciate in your life—

friends, family, your health, your body, spiritual qualities, even material things. There are no wrong answers. We recommend writing your list rather than simply making it in your head, but doing it mentally is better than not doing it at all. Some of our students have exercised their creativity in making their gratitude lists; we've seen poems and drawings of people's favorite things. The more you acknowledge and pay attention to positive things, the more you value and appreciate those things, and the better you tend to feel about yourself and your life—and a happier person is a more attractive person!

⤳ *Chapter Highlights*

♦ A woman makes the first move by being attractive. A man must make the next move by doing something to show he is interested.

♦ Unfortunately, there are only frogs out there, so a woman must make her white knight out of one of them.

♦ When a woman who is hunting spots an enthusiastic man, she may work her turn-on by dangling some bait, like a smile, a wink, or a glance.

♦ Have enough confidence to get out there and take some swings. Being rejected at least proves that you're playing the game.

CHAPTER 2

You're the jewel in my crown,

You allow me to clown.

The time to my clock,

You're the key to my lock.

Pillow Talk Plus

Tips on Communication

*M*en and boys are still brought up to see themselves as valued for their abilities to produce and get things done, and women and girls are still brought up to be valued for their abilities to attract and consume. This doesn't mean that women aren't interested in being productive or that men aren't concerned with being attractive. We're talking in general terms about traits that have been very successfully ingrained in the two sexes over many centuries of societal conditioning. This difference—men as producers and doers and women as attractors and consumers—can be the cause of both much of the fun that happens when women and men get together and of a lot of the pain that we can choose to take on when relating to members of the other sex.

Anthropologists and sociologists have theories about the origins of these characteristics. According to Helen Fisher and other scholars, thousands of years ago female humans who were able to get the best food for themselves and their offspring were the ones who survived and thrived and lived to bear more offspring. Thus, back when sex roles dictated that men were the hunters and women were the tenders of the hearth, women looked for mates who could provide well for them. Evolution favored these traits. Over countless generations, then, human females evolved into beings that are good at wanting things and human males into beings that are good at obtaining goals.

When you put the two together you have the possibility for something that is greater than the sum of the parts. Men live to succeed in meeting their mates' desires. Women want lots of attention and they want material objects, things that will make them feel more attractive. This is why when you look in my closet you will find about four pairs of shoes, three of them sneakers, and when you look in Vera's closet you will find perhaps fifty pairs of shoes, two of them sneakers. Whether the evolutionary argument offered by these scholars is accurate is still debatable. What is not debatable is that most stores and catalogs cater to women more than they do to men.

This chapter discusses how a man can give a woman the attention she craves, and how a woman can encourage a man in his efforts to please her. It also addresses how both sexes can play—and win—the game of seduction.

❦ Noticing and Paying Attention ❦

Men like to use logic and to follow rules and formulas when dealing with anything. However, no exact formula applies when relating to a woman. When it comes to dealing with women, it is more important to keep your attention on her and to keep your options open than to stick to any rules. When your attention is focused on her and you remain flexible in your responses, you are able to notice whether you are getting closer to her or moving farther away. You can tell whether she likes your attention, is overwhelmed, or is just not very interested, and you can tailor your next moves accordingly.

Use your senses to notice how a woman responds to your attentions. This works whether you are trying to pick her up for the first time or have been together for many years. In longtime relationships, people often start taking the other person for granted and stop noticing her or him. Look at a woman's eyes and face to observe whether she is lighting up or fading away. People are not difficult to read if you can remove your attention from yourself and from the chronic inner recitation of prejudices and doubts that so many of us seem to engage in. Simply place your attention on the other person and notice the effects of your doing so.

Another way to sense where a woman's interest is directed is to notice your own feelings and sensations as you interact with her. If your feelings and her responses are positive—if you sense that you're winning and you observe her eyes shining brightly, for example—then continue with what you are doing. If, on the other hand, you feel negative, like someone said or did something to offend you, even if you cannot pinpoint the exact source of the attack, it is a good sign that you are meeting resistance. In this case it is time to change tactics and try a different approach. Women have been conditioned, probably forever, to resist male attention in one way or another. Yet most women also have a strong natural desire to receive male attention. Therein lies the conflict—and also an opportunity. Use this discrepancy to get closer to her and get to know her better.

A woman who is interested in a man wants his full attention, or at least his willingness to give it to her. Especially when they are first going out, she wants to feel that she is the most important thing he has to focus on. She wants him to be interested in her and not be looking around at other women or talking on his cell phone. Women are satiable, both sexually and otherwise, and once a woman realizes that a man is eager to give her all of his attention, she usually becomes willing to share it with other things.

∾ What to Say ∾

As we've said, there are no specific guidelines or formulas to follow when interacting with a woman. It is helpful to know that women love to be flattered, to be told how beautiful they are, and to be appreciated and approved of. Men like to hear these things too, but it seems less important to them than it does to women. Furthermore, men like compliments to be more specific. Whereas a woman loves hearing how wonderful she is, most men would prefer to hear exactly *how* they were wonderful: for example, "You were wonderful in how you handled your brother's anger over his wife's lateness."

To some extent, this holds true for women, too. Even though they love to be flattered in a general way, it is more seductive and shows that you're really paying attention if you can be specific. Let her know how beautifully her hair glistens in the sunlight or how great she smells. Tell her how radiantly and stunningly her eyes sparkle when she smiles. Tell her what wonderful, soft, silky skin she has. Vera says that almost every woman thinks her thighs are wrong, even though lots of men like and are attracted to lots of women's thighs of all shapes and sizes. Maybe one woman in ten thousand believes that her thighs are just right. If you find yourself in a situation where you can compliment a woman on her beautiful thighs, you will win favor with her.

Flattery and compliments can certainly be more than skin deep. Anything positive about a woman is worth appreciating and acknowledging. If you like her sense of humor, let her know. When she demonstrates being kind and having a good heart, show her that you noticed and appreciate it. If she is smart or a good decorator, point out the pleasure this brings to your life.

This will work with anyone, not only women, because approval and acknowledgment are the best tools we have for getting closer to another human being. (And, as sort of a bonus, showing our appreciation to others is also one of the best ways to increase our appreciation of our own lives.) Be sincere, and don't overdo it. If a person doesn't like themselves very much and you go overboard flattering them, they will think either that you want something from them or that you are crazy. By noticing if your compliments and flatteries charm the other person or cause them to move away from you, you will know when it is time to stop and when to continue.

Women, it's useful to know that men live to succeed. Their ultimate goal is to win, especially with a woman. Many women fail to acknowledge their men, who will do almost anything to get some approval. A woman can get a man to do her bidding by verbally appreciating what he does for her or to her, and her doing so will probably make him even more productive. A woman needn't lavish a whole lot of praise on a man to be more approving than many other women; knowing this and acting on it are the keys to attracting and keeping a good man. Vera helped me to become a successful writer through her positive reinforcement. I never believed I could write very well, so I took mostly math and science courses in college to avoid having to write term papers. Vera read some little thing I once wrote and told me how much she enjoyed it. From then on, every time I wrote something, whether it was a poem, a story, or an essay, she encouraged and complimented me on how well it was written and how much pleasure she got from reading it. Both men and women can benefit from the exercise on verbal appreciation that we've included at the end of this chapter.

Some men have difficulty saying "I love you." They believe they are demonstrating their love just by being there. In truth, the nicer and more romantic a man is and the more sweet-talking he does (within limits of course; a woman won't trust a guy who is always sweet-talking her), the better his odds are in his quest to go to bed with a woman. This means that if he really feels love for her (and *only* if he really feels it), he should say so. It does not mean he should tell her he loves her on their first date. Obviously, his doing so wouldn't be seductive even if it were true. He must be selective with his compliments and also must notice whether they are being received with delight or with an indication that the woman isn't yet ready to go there. Flirting involves noticing and appreciating yourself, and perhaps someone else, as a sexual being, and sending signals to show those feelings. The intensity of the sexual signal can fall anywhere on the spectrum from friendly and light to erotically strong. Flirting is a two-way street, and if nothing is being returned it is a signal to back off.

∾ Listening to (and Interpreting) Womanese ∾

Many women, both those in relationships and those who are looking for one, often complain that men do not listen to what they are saying. By becoming a good listener a man can gain points with women and can move to the head of the suitor line. Being a good listener is part of the attention that is so critical in getting to know someone and growing closer to her. Make eye contact when you're in conversation with a woman or listening to her responses. Your eye contact needn't be constant—you don't want to make her uncomfortable— just enough to show your interest. Respond to what she says with a nod or other acknowledgment that indicates you've heard her. Phrases like "aha," "right," "I see," "yes," or even "wow" show her that you are listening. Do not interrupt while she is talking. Wait till she pauses, and, when it is appropriate or when you require more information, ask questions about what she has said that could lead to further disclosure of her feelings and thoughts.

Even though men and women from the same country speak the same tongue, the two sexes have a slightly different language. Many men find it difficult to follow what a woman is saying or what she is actually asking for. The highest and best gift you can give a woman is your full attention. Women often just want to talk and express their feelings, but frequently, when a man hears his woman express some complaint or want, his immediate response is to wonder what he can do to remedy the situation, help her to feel better, or make her happy.

I have made this mistake more than once with Vera. Often, when she simply wanted to express her desires or to discuss our goals and for me to listen, my response has been to assume that her telling me these things was a request for action, that she wanted me to do or say something to make things all right. We went through one of these episodes recently. We live in a lovely little apartment where we have been very happy for ten years. Recently, a larger apartment on the upper floor became available. Vera began talking to me about possibly moving to the larger place. I immediately concluded that she was no longer happy in our apartment and began to get in a bad frame of mind about moving. I took it upon myself to go see the place, try to figure out what to do, make some decisions, talk to the landlord, and do whatever was necessary to fix the situation. I discovered that the new apartment would be quite hot in the summertime and got even more bummed about having to make the change. Meanwhile, Vera only wanted to fantasize about moving. She never seriously wanted to move, and here I was jumping through all these hoops that turned out to be unnecessary. To make it easier for the man and have him respond how she wants him to, a woman can start a conversation by telling him she just wants to talk about some things and is not looking for him to remedy the situation or present any solutions yet. Then he will know to alter his normal fix-it behavior and will respond appropriately.

Another example of a woman's seeming to ask for one thing and actually wanting something else occurred when our friends John and Mary lived in a home where their bedroom faced south. The bedroom got very hot in the summertime from the sun's beating directly on the window. Mary kept telling John she wanted to get thick draperies for the window in that room. He didn't understand her request because the room was very small and thick draperies wouldn't fit with the design of the rest of the room. Finally he understood that what she really wanted was for the bedroom to be cooler, so he had an air conditioner installed. This took care of the hot room, and Mary stopped asking for thick draperies and chose more delicate ones.

Women also tend to speak more randomly than men. When a number of women are together they may jump quickly from one topic to another and have no difficulty following the conversation. If you were to introduce a man into this mix, he may have a difficult time following the flow of the conversation as it would appear to him to lack logical "bridges" between the various topics. He may get lost and miss a lot of what is being said. When a woman wants to get her point and ideas across to a man, she is well advised to slow down and keep to the issue at hand and let him know when she is going to change topics.

Women sometimes complain that men do not express themselves often enough or deeply enough. Women will talk to each other for long periods of time about their feelings and desires. Because of this conditioning that allows women to open up with each other, when they are with a man, they may think he is holding back. If a man can get past the conditioning that tells him to keep his feelings to himself, and if he can learn to express himself more, he will be on his way to creating a better rapport with the women in his life. The more open and expressive a man can be about his desires, the more open the woman he is with will be about her real desires without having to edit or censor them. If he is unable to do this, then at least by asking a woman questions about herself and her desires he can show that he is interested in her and in her likes and dislikes.

When listening to a woman, it is a good idea occasionally to bring up something analogous in your life, so she does not think she is on the hot seat, but bring the focus back to her when you feel she is ready for more attention. We have met many women who have dumped a man because on their first date all he did was talk about himself—his life, his past and future goals, his story. It is okay to talk about yourself to some extent, but people will be more fascinated with you if you focus your attention on them and show interest in their story. Notice how often you use the word "I"; if it keeps coming up, you are probably being self-absorbed.

∾ Admit when It Hurts ∾

Besides failing to acknowledge the good and wonderful things a woman does and how she adds to their lives, many men also fail to mention when they feel hurt. Lots of men think they're supposed to be tough and that tough guys do not let on when they're hurt. This may be effective in war and in some sports; however, when relating to a woman, a refusal to admit that what she said or did bothered you or had any effect on you will often result in her feeling unnoticed by you. Again, being noticed is extremely important to women. Your acting as if you did not feel anything could cause her to believe that she has had no effect on you. In such a case she may raise the ante to see if you will notice the next, more hurtful thing she says or does.

This does not mean you have to whine or complain over every little thing that happens to you; most women do not find men who bitch a lot very attractive. Indeed, some women believe they have the exclusive rights to bitching. However, when a woman is causing you pain—whether she appears to be doing it deliberately or otherwise—it will be beneficial for you to at least say "ouch." Then you can find out what she wants, what is frustrating her, or what you have done that is producing her unkind behavior. It may turn out to have nothing to do with you. Perhaps someone at work or elsewhere dissed her or treated her cruelly or made a sexist remark. In some ways it can be a good thing that she is taking it out on you; that means she feels close enough to you and safe enough with you to be mean to you. You are the man on whom she has chosen to take out her frustrations; you are responsible for all the male-chauvinist attitudes she comes up against. Nevertheless, in as nice a way as you can, let her know when she touches a nerve. The sooner you communicate with her and express your painful feelings, the better will be your frame of mind. If you let your resentment linger without mentioning it, as more pain comes your way you will handle it with less and less grace. The spring-cleaning exercise at the end of Chapter 4 can be a very helpful tool for keeping your mind free of old pains.

∼ What Not to Say ∼

Vera and I were having lunch with an acquaintance recently who joked that Vera had the beginnings of a potbelly. Even though it was said in jest, those are stupid words for a man to ever use with a woman. One time when I was about twenty years old and engaged to my first wife, I teasingly called her tubby. I thought the comment was cute at the time, but she got very mad at me and stayed that way for practically the whole summer. She nearly called our wedding off. Women are valued in our society for being attractive, and our society equates fat with ugly. Therefore, any word like *fat, tubby, large, big,* etc., will immediately cause most women to "lose" (i.e., to feel bad or like a loser)—and to get angry with whoever said it. So even if you're tempted to say it because you think it's cute or funny, take some advice and never use any variation of the f-word around a woman.

As we described in Chapter 1, women test men—continually, it seems to some men—and one of the tests that is a setup for potential failure is when she asks you if she looks fat in a certain outfit, for example, "Does this dress make me look fat?" The answer to that question is either "no" or "no way." If she responds by saying she thinks it *does* make her look fat, do not respond and do not argue. She has not asked you for any more information, and you do not want to get into that area unless you are her doctor or diet coach, which is not a job for someone's husband or lover.

Any other references to a woman's being unattractive are foolish things for a man to say, in earnest or in jest. Do not tell her she looks tired, wrinkled, horrible, witchy, dreadful—or anything else that sounds like "ugly." Vera and I play a little game wherein if one of us is frowning or looking unhappy the other reminds that person to smile. This usually works, and besides feeling better the person looks better, too. It may be okay at certain times to tell a woman that her behavior or actions are repulsive or ugly, but even in this context it is probably wise to choose different words. Good communication usually means saying how *you* feel in relation to what she said or did—that you feel hurt, for example, or that her actions upset you. This is good advice for both men and women. Keeping the focus on yourself when describing your feelings of hurt or anger is better than saying negative things about your partner. Name-calling will never get you points with anyone. To call another person, especially someone close to you and whom you supposedly love, stupid or an idiot or ugly will only cause that person to resent you and want to hurt you back or to leave you—not a good idea if you want to go to bed with that person.

We knew a sweet woman who had a bad habit of misplacing her keys, wallet, purse, or whatever she was carrying. Whenever her husband found out about her losing something, he would get mad and call her all kinds of mean names. She felt bad enough herself for having lost the item, and his added insults did nothing to help her. She ended up leaving him (true to her nature, she "lost" him too) and eventually married a much mellower guy. Her new husband's approach was to help her find the misplaced item, and when he did, she appreciated and acknowledged him as her hero. Instead of both partners feeling terrible, the couple created a fun game out of this potentially negative situation. They are totally devoted to each other and have a lot of fun together, and the guy gets to be a hero instead of being angry.

Men also have their soft spots and susceptibilities. Because men tend to be production-oriented, saying anything to imply that a man is a failure or is impotent will cause his ego to cringe. Furthermore, most men are totally hexed by penis size, even though as we point out in Chapter 6, "Her Side of the

Bed," it really is not a vital issue when it comes to producing pleasure for a woman who has a turned-on clitoris. More on that topic later.

∼ Lack of Communication ∼

We knew a husband and wife who seemed to be quite in love with each other. They both worked, and the woman also went to school. Because of their busy schedules they did not see each other very much. In the early stages of their relationship the husband never seemed to look at other women; he only had eyes for his wife. However, after the woman was out of school and they were spending more time together, he began to notice and make comments about attractive women that happened to pass by. This really perturbed his wife because she thought he was going to leave her for another woman. This went on for a couple of years until she finally left him due to his roving eye.

This story is a tragedy that did not have to unfold as it did. It basically arose from a lack of communication between the two people that allowed them to create their own narrow viewpoints about what the other person was doing and thinking. Most men notice and are attracted to women who pass by them in their everyday lives. Thus, for this couple the first lie that flourished was that early in their relationship the man did not notice other women. Then when he started to admit that he was noticing other attractive women, his wife went crazy because she had been led to believe that he was not interested in anyone else, and now all of a sudden he was. Perhaps she felt less attractive as she grew older. She also had more time once she finished school to concern herself with what her husband was doing. Whatever the combination of things that caused it, she was led to believe that other, younger women were putting the make on her man and that he was responding to them. Instead, she could have realized that she was still beautiful and that she had the power to have her husband be loyal to her. She could have appreciated the fact that he was finally telling the truth when he admitted noticing other pretty women. This could have been an opportunity for them to become closer to each other.

When Vera and I are on one of our many walks, we cross paths with lots of sexy and pretty women and girls. It is fun to communicate to her what I like about them—their nice legs or shapely butt or great hair. Vera will make observations back to me, either agreeing with my taste or letting me know that she thinks they have too much cellulite or whatever. She will even point out an attractive woman if for some reason I missed her. Vera knows I am not going to leave her just because some woman has a great butt, nor does she feel less attractive because of my roving eye. Men tend to look at other women; it's just a fact. At the same time, a man will benefit from noticing his partner and complimenting her whenever she looks good or dresses up. When a woman feels attractive and knows that her partner finds her so, she will not get so bent out of shape when he notices other pretty women.

Besides just looking good, there are some sexy women out there, thank goodness, who have some turn-on and are willing to let the world feel it. Sometimes a man is sexually turned on by a woman, maybe even someone he has seen on television. This does not mean he is going to chase her or ask her to bed. He may not even realize who caused this reaction. He can use the energy from his turn-on to romance his partner and seduce her into bed. His partner may or may not respond to his desire. If she does, that's great; if she doesn't, it could be a good time for him to masturbate. We think masturbation is a useful and appropriate response to sexual turn-on. We have known a number of couples who would get into fights because the man wanted to have sex and the woman did not. He would get pissed at her, feel rejected, and blow off steam by picking a fight rather than using the energy as fuel for his pleasure. Instead of fighting with his partner, a man in that situation has a number of pleasurable options: He can play with her resistance and use his seductive skills to change her mind, or he can adjourn to the bedroom and have a great time with himself.

Some couples can live together, not talk to each other often, and still have a decent marriage. There are all kinds of folks out there and if two people can be in agreement about not talking, then it may work for them. However, we wouldn't call this arrangement a fantastic marriage. In order for a partnership to be fantastic, communication must be current, flowing, and kind. Each person does what it takes to learn about their partner. They will know about each other's past, desires and goals, likes and dislikes, and everything else they can discover. This is what intimacy is: the union of two different people into one strong unit. Each person will be there for the other when he or she is down and needs a shoulder to rest on. Each person will take their partner's side in practically all instances. In many bad marriages when one person is down, the other says things to keep them there or to make them feel even worse. In a good marriage if one person is down, the other is up and helps the partner get back up by reassuring him or her that he or she is a good, wonderful, and right person. When I get down, Vera is always there to tell me that I—or, usually, that *we*—can handle everything and it's going to be okay. I feel her support and as a result don't stay down very long.

∼ Appetite and Production ∼

As we've discussed, in our society much of a woman's value is based on her attractiveness (which doesn't mean she has to have classic movie-star beauty), and her attractiveness is inseparable from her appetite. By contrast, men in our society are valued more for their productive abilities. This does not mean that men cannot be attractive and want things, or that women cannot be productive, only that our society values one trait for men and the other for women with much greater emphasis. A woman who displays genuine appetite and who consumes with passion is attractive both to men and to other women. Women may seek her out and try to imitate her behavior. When a man finds a woman with an authentic appetite for something, he wants to fill her up till she is stuffed. This is true both because real desire has a magnetic effect on people and also because it presents an opportunity for the man to show off his productive talents.

This value system also accounts for why women want to appear insatiable. On one level, if a woman were to admit to being satisfied, she might feel as though she is no longer attractive. In her mind her value is connected with her ability to consume, and if she is filled up then she is unable to consume any more. This of course is not true. Women *are* satiable, and a woman who is fully gratified is most attractive. She glows from the pleasurable attention and swallows the experience with much appreciation. We include more information on the myth of women's insatiability in Chapter 7, "His Side of the Bed."

Let us clarify that when we talk about women as consumers, we are not equating that with being a shopaholic. Authentic appetite often has to do with things that are unrelated to material goods. Indeed, an unquenchable need to accumulate more and more "stuff" can indicate that a person is discontented with himself or herself, which, as we've discussed, is the opposite of attractive. A woman can express desire for many different things and experiences: a day spent in nature, time to devote to a hobby or passion, a sensuous evening of lovemaking, a delightful meal prepared by her beloved, a good workout. Yet sometimes an elegant new dress or a new pair of shoes is just what she wants. True appetite is when a person enjoys what they already have as well as what they receive. It is not about getting things just to get them. A woman who enjoys whatever she has or is presented with is a pleasure for anyone to produce for.

For that matter, a woman can buy her own diamond rings or give herself an orgasm. To create a good life doesn't require having a partner. In fact, a mediocre relationship and a mediocre sex life aren't any better than being alone. We do believe, however, that a great relationship makes life more fun. A sunset shared with a loved one seems more beautiful than one seen alone. A shared meal or an orgasm produced by someone who knows you and your body is more pleasurable than one experienced alone.

There are three major components to appetite. The first is the raw desire, the craving, the wanting, the yearning, the aspiring for a sensation, a material thing, or an experience. The second is the meeting of the desire, the filling up of the craving, or the realization of the aspiration. The final ingredient is the swallowing, the digestion, the appreciation, the acknowledgment. This last component is often overlooked and underused. If a person doesn't swallow, they will fill up very fast. If they take the next bite without having swallowed the last, they will be unable to assimilate it and will have to spit it out, so to speak.

How does one develop this aspect of appetite? Sometimes simply saying some words of appreciation and acknowledging that one is full are enough to allow one to consume more. (We explore acknowledgment further in Chapter 6, "Her Side of the Bed.") On other occasions it may be best to allow some time before taking the next bite. When a man gives a woman more experiences or material goods than she can consume, the experiences will go downhill and the objects will turn into garbage.

Another way of swallowing or appreciating something is to share it with others who have more use for it than you. By giving away your surplus, you free yourself to have more. The goal of giving is best served by taking pleasure in the giving itself rather than doing it to buy friendship or votes or loyalty or prestige or for any self-serving reason other than because it feels good.

False appetite and poor digestion (for example, forgetting to swallow) are sources of misery and pain. Real desire is a beautiful thing to behold and is the source of much happiness.

∾ Seduction ∾

According to Robert Greene, in *The Art of Seduction*, the Latin root word for *seduce* means to lead astray. If you think about it, seduction of another person involves getting them to do something or to go somewhere that they had not originally intended—in other words, to go astray. In *The Art of Seduction*, a book we highly recommend, Mr. Greene outlines ten basic personality types—such as "siren," "rake," "gentle charmer," and "natural," for example—and describes how each person can access the qualities inherent in his or her type to become the best seducer possible. (He calls the tenth type the "antiseducer.") Both men and women can be the seducer or the seduced.

The basic difference between a seducer (no matter which type) and an antiseducer is that good seducers have developed the ability to place a lot of attention on someone else. They are focused on the person they are seducing; they are pleasure-oriented and can draw the object of their seduction into that pleasure. (We know that the word *object* can have negative connotations in the context of sexuality and relationships. We intend no such meaning here.) By contrast, the antiseducer is self-absorbed, insecure, and unable to place much attention on anyone outside of himself or herself. Antiseducers never realize when they are pestering, imposing, or talking too much.

Mr. Greene also identifies eighteen types of "victims" of seduction, including, for example, the aging baby, the rescuer, the lonely leader, and the sensualist. (Again, we don't use the word *victim* here in a negative sense. To be a "pleasure victim" is actually to reach the highest possible state of pleasure; it is to be someone who is willing to surrender to pleasure. This means letting another person take control of your senses. For an example of how this might work from a gastronomic standpoint, imagine eating a dish that has been prepared by someone else and that you have never tried before. You find it delicious. You have temporarily trusted your senses to the chef. Sexually speaking, to be a pleasure victim means to allow someone else to take you for a sensual ride. The downside is that surrendering to pleasure can feel risky and to some extent can leave one vulnerable. However, a person can only reach the highest levels of sensation when he or she totally surrenders, and a good seducer enables his or her "victim" to trust that it is okay to do so. (For more on the topic of being a pleasure victim, see Chapter 8.) Whether there are eighteen or one hundred types of pleasure victims, each person is unique and must be treated so. The better a seducer understands his or her intended victim, the better he or she can plan the seduction.

So what are some general strategies for seduction? Instead of using a direct approach, sometimes it works better to go slowly and take your time getting to know someone. If possible, find out as much as you can beforehand about your intended "seducee." The more information you have, the better you will be able to plan your seduction. If you have mutual friends, ask them where this person likes to go and what he or she likes to do. Then, you can show up at some of the places where they go, but do not confront them directly at first; approach them "from an angle," as Mr. Greene says. Get fairly close but not too close. Maybe place yourself in the person's vicinity for a short time and then remove yourself from his or her viewing area. You do not want to appear as though you are stalking them; this is a definite turn-off and will ruin your plan. A woman can dress seductively to get a man's attention, and then disappear from his view and suddenly reappear.

I love the movie *Groundhog Day* because Bill Murray's character has to relive the same day over and over. At first he uses this newfound power—or punishment, as he sees it—to exploit people. Then he tries to kill himself a number of times and even fails at that. Things start working out for him when he uses his strange condition to fall in love with and to seduce Rita, who is wonderfully acted by Andie McDowell. He uses each day to discover more about her: what she likes and dislikes, her favorite foods and music, even what she likes to say as a toast when she has a drink. He finds out she likes French poetry, so he learns French and memorizes poetry and recites it to her. She likes musicians, so he becomes a virtuoso pianist. Meanwhile he also performs all kinds of good deeds, such as saving lives and preventing accidents, and is transformed from a schmuck into a wonderful human being. You won't have as much time as this guy does to investigate your target or get as many opportunities to learn from your mistakes, but if you study and plan your strategy carefully, you will have more confidence when you finally meet your intended victim. If you make mistakes that ruin your chances, use them constructively, learn from them, and apply the lessons to your next act of seduction.

The most important thing is to enjoy whatever you are doing. If a certain activity feels like it is too much work and not worth the bother, then maybe you shouldn't be doing it. However, if you are enjoying yourself, even if some occasional doubt creeps up about the value and significance of what you are doing, do not let it stop you. Continue with your seduction.

As we've discussed, it is a good idea to compliment and flatter your victim. But when does flattery turn into pestering? How do you know when you have crossed the line and gone too far? At what point does your appreciation for someone turn into an imposition? These are all valid questions. The answers will make themselves evident when you keep your attention on the other person. In general, it is best to stop before they have had enough in order to leave them wanting more. This is true both in seduction and also when sexually gratifying someone. By looking at the person's face and reading his or her body language—and also by noticing how your own body feels—you can tell if he or she is still receptive to you, is starting to go away, or is simply less receptive than before. As soon as you notice this occurring, stop pulling the person toward you and instead begin to push him or her away. Push as far as is necessary; hopefully only a little pushing will cause him or her to come toward you again. If you waited too long to start pushing, you may have to push farther than if you had noticed earlier.

What do we mean by "push him or her away"? How does one do this effectively? A friend of ours liked a man who lived more than an hour away from her. They had a date planned, but he was making noises like he wanted to back out because he had to work the next day. She wanted him to come to her. She wanted to be his priority. But she told him over the phone that he should not to come see her that night. She told him it was time for them to take a break. She told him not even to call her until he was ready to decide that having fun with her would make his life better. He showed up that night.

We had another friend who as a young woman visited Rome. She met a cute Italian guy who asked her out to dinner. She said yes, thinking he would take her to a charming local restaurant. They got into his car, and all of a sudden they were leaving Rome, heading for the suburbs. She asked where he was going. He said he planned to fix dinner for her at his home. She gave him a look of disapproval, so he immediately swung the car around and headed back to her hotel. As soon as he did, she thought, "He is willing to do what I ask so quickly; maybe dinner at his place would be all right." So she changed her mind, went with him to his home, and enjoyed a great dinner that night and great sex for the rest of the time she was in Rome.

The bottom line is that the seducer must focus his or her attention on the seducee at all times in order to figure out when to show interest and when to leave or back off. The seducer must learn—sometimes through trial and error—when to be nice and when to push the other person away. The seducer must tune in to determine when the opportune time presents itself to get the other person into bed and create outrageous pleasure together.

One of the tricks of seduction is to approach and retreat and approach and retreat. First you start with a pleasurable offer. For example, I might ask Vera to go to bed so I can ravish her. If she looks like she is resisting, then I might "retreat" by saying something like, "You just look so beautiful that I got carried away. I know we have to get some work done first on our book because the publisher has a deadline. However, we work better after we have had some orgasmic pleasure, so maybe we should have pleasure first. Then again, it *is* early in the day, and we had fun last night, so maybe it's too soon. On the other hand, the more we make love, the more you enjoy it. Then again, I don't think you're only about sex and lust, so maybe we could just talk. Or maybe we could talk and have orgasmic pleasure at the same time. . . ." You get the idea. You want to keep your intended victim off balance so they are unable to predict what you are going to do next.

Being too interested and too attentive is a turn-off to many people. People like to be liked, but if you like them more than they can handle, they often seem to think something is wrong with you for liking them so much. This was the case with a friend of ours whenever he dated someone new. Things would usually start off well; the two would enjoy each other and have good times together. The problem came when the woman wanted to get closer and hinted that maybe she'd like to move in with him. Regardless if he was the one who initially chased her, this little bit of closeness and positive attention from a woman would send him running in the opposite direction. Like Groucho Marx, our friend didn't want to join any club that would have him for a member. Most people are not as extreme as this fellow; still, it is a good idea to notice how much positive attention your seducee can handle. By not always being available, you will cause your target to want more from you. This goes for both sexes. As we stated in the previous chapter, a woman who appears too needy and clingy has the effect of repulsing most men.

Women can be very powerful seducers. By carefully selecting her words, actions, costumes, and innuendos a woman can get a man to do almost anything. Cleopatra is one of the best-known seducers of all time, male or female. She used her turn-on combined with her wits to make men bend over backward for her. A woman has the added advantage of being able to turn a guy on and compel him to come toward her without even having to say anything. To tap into this potential she must like herself and be aware of her power over men. A woman who is too aggressive may turn some guys off, so she has to know what kind of man she is dealing with by first paying him some attention. Some men appreciate an aggressive woman who knows and asks for what she wants. When she adds her turn-on, such a man will become her "sex slave" or whatever else she may want him to be. Other men either may be afraid of an aggressive woman or may want to be the aggressor themselves and therefore will not respond to the direct approach. Even in these cases a woman can use her turn-on and cause her target to think he is the one seducing her. She can lure him into her trap without his ever realizing she is doing so. In the old days a woman would drop her handkerchief near a man whom she wanted to seduce so he could pick it up and return it to her. And we've all seen movies in which a woman feigns hurting her ankle so the man she's after will help her. Women can use all kinds of tricks to get a man to assist them.

A not uncommon response once a seduction has been successfully accomplished is for one or both parties to lose interest in the pursuit or to feel somewhat let down because the chase is over. These are natural feelings, and you can respond by either continuing the relationship or moving on to a fresh target. If you wish to continue with the relationship, either party can start a new series of seductive moves, backing away and then returning, etc. Sometimes the roles will switch, and the original seducer will become the seducee and vice versa. As long as you are having fun with the seduction you can use variations on the push/pull technique no matter what stage your relationship is in. The better you know each other, however, the more you may have to refine the technique and be clever in how you use it, because your partner may figure out what you're up to. Remember, too, that a woman can always use her turn-on to get a man to respond to her.

Another option is to continue to get to know the other person by exposing more of who you are and discovering more about who the other person is. A third option you can use to keep a relationship thrilling is to explore techniques designed to enhance pleasure and orgasmic possibility, such as those we teach. These strategies aren't mutually exclusive. Most highly successful long-term relationships use some combination of these and other tactics to keep things hot over the years.

In the next chapter, "Who Makes the Bed?" we discuss the fact that in the best relationships the participants give to each other because they enjoy giving rather than because they're looking for something in return. We also discuss other roles and responsibilities in the relationship. After that, Chapter 4, "Getting Ready for Bed," explores the insidiousness of anger and its harmful effects on pleasure.

✧ EXERCISE 2A ✧
Verbal Appreciation

Verbally expressing your appreciation to others not only makes them feel good; the greatest reward lies in how good and how much more appreciative of your own life doing so will make you feel. Some of you may already express your appreciation to others regularly, in which case you will find it easy to do this simple exercise. All that is required is to say something nice to your partner at least once a day. If you don't have a partner, say something nice at least once a day to someone you come into contact with. It can be anyone you wish—stranger, acquaintance, or good friend. When expressing appreciation to a man, acknowledge something he has done or how good he makes you feel. The more specific the compliment, the better. Instead of saying, "You are such a great guy," say, "I really appreciate it that you fixed the leak in the bathroom sink today," or whatever. When appreciating a woman, you can notice how attractive she is—including complimenting her clothes, shoes, hair, body, or face—or you can acknowledge a behavior or character trait you admire, such as her sense of humor or honesty. Again, it helps to be specific. If you praise someone other than your partner, make sure your compliments will not be confused with sexual harassment. Offering verbal appreciation to others will cause you to feel better about yourself; in turn, you'll also be amazed at how people will appreciate you more.

✧ EXERCISE 2B ✧
Look and Touch

This is a simple yet effective communication exercise that involves learning to ask for something you want. Two people sit facing each other on the floor or bed, with clothes on or off. One person is the coach and the other is the student. The student begins by making eye contact with the coach, and then asking if he or she may look at a specific part of the coach's body—for example, "May I look at your right elbow?" The coach responds with a yes or a no. Whatever the answer is, the student replies by saying, "Thank you." If the answer is yes, the student looks at the coach's right elbow for a few seconds, enjoying the experience as much as he or she can. The student finishes by again saying, "Thank you." Then the student asks the coach if he or she may touch a specific body part—for example, "May I touch your left elbow?" The coach responds with a yes or a no. The student thanks the coach for either answer. If the answer is yes, the student touches the coach's left elbow with one hand. The student simply feels the elbow with as much pleasure as he or she can, without rubbing or stroking. After a few seconds the student removes the hand and again says thank you.

If the coach says yes, he or she makes it easy for the student to look at or touch the body part in question. For example, if the student asks to look at the coach's back, the coach turns around to show his or her back. The coach also focuses on the body part being looked at or touched and allows it to feel as pleasurable as possible. We recommend that the coach respond occasionally with a no so the student can overcome feeling rejected and hopefully ask again later to look at or touch the same body part. It is okay for the student to ask to look at or touch the coach's genitals or other erogenous areas. As usual, the coach can say either yes or no. Do the exercise for a few minutes and then switch roles.

◡ *Chapter Highlights*

- ◆ Approval and acknowledgment are the best tools we have for getting closer to another human being. They also help us to appreciate our own lives.

- ◆ A woman needn't lavish a whole lot of praise on a man to be more approving than many other women; knowing that and acting on it are the keys to attracting and keeping a good man.

- ◆ Women often just want to talk and express their feelings, but frequently, when a man hears his woman express some complaint or want, his immediate response is to wonder what he can do to remedy the situation, help her to feel better, or make her happy.

- ◆ Women who display genuine appetite and who consume with passion are attractive to men and to other women.

- ◆ A woman who enjoys whatever she has or is presented with is a pleasure for anyone to produce for.

- ◆ By giving away your surplus, you free yourself up to have more.

- ◆ A person can only reach the highest levels of sensation when he or she totally surrenders, and a good seducer enables his or her "pleasure victim" to trust that it is okay to do so.

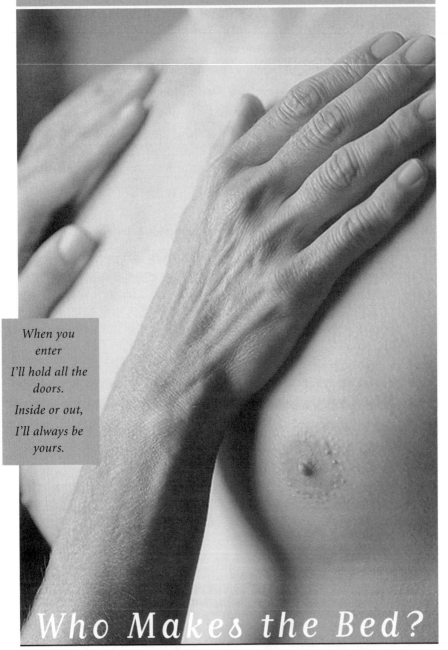

CHAPTER 3

When you
enter
I'll hold all the
doors.
Inside or out,
I'll always be
yours.

Who Makes the Bed?

Roles and Responsibilities
in a Relationship

*T*his chapter can be thought of as a primer of sorts on how to create a successful intimate partnership. It addresses responsibilities shared by both partners as well as men's and women's separate roles. We include this topic because gender roles are much less defined than they used to be, yet, as should be evident from what we've written so far in this book, we believe that the differences between men and women lead to some natural division of relationship skills. The chapter concludes with an introductory discussion of sexual satisfaction.

～ Nonreciprocity, or Don't Keep Score ～

A successful intimate relationship cannot depend on reciprocity—that is, on keeping score. This is the opposite of how friendships operate. Friends usually take turns doing favors for one another or paying for outings, and they try to keep the balance as even as possible. By contrast, if two lovers keep score of who did what for whom and how much was given and who owes more, then the relationship is doomed. This goes for everything, from taking out the garbage to bestowing back rubs to giving and receiving sensual pleasure. Intimate relationships work best when both partners put in as much as they can without waiting for the other to reciprocate before they put in more. You can think of it as each party giving 100 percent instead of trying to negotiate a fifty-fifty contract. A relationship will not survive a tit-for-tat mentality. The more unconditionally each partner's love is given, the greater the chance that the relationship will blossom.

We do not mean to suggest that it does not matter what the other person is doing or how they feel about the one who is giving 100 percent. If the second party is not in love with, is not interested in a relationship with, or couldn't care less about the first party, then no matter how much unconditional love is given, no relationship exists. In such a case, if it makes you feel good to continue to give unconditionally, even if nothing is coming back, then carry on with this behavior. However, most people will feel better and will be mentally healthier when their giving is at least appreciated by the other person and when some care is returned. We have known some women and even a few men who totally served their spouses and received hardly anything in return. This is not a relationship, and unless a person is in agreement with this arrangement, they must stand up for themselves and say, "Enough!" When either member of a relationship feels they are not getting theirs, it is time to have a discussion, to ask each other some questions, or to bring in outside help. The sooner one acts on these feelings, the easier the road will be to feeling better.

I was once madly in love with a girl who seemed to like me but didn't return any of the passionate feelings I had for her. I wrote her poetry and gave her flowers and gifts, but she hardly responded. I enjoyed this crush and the chance to open myself romantically, but after a number of months it dawned on me that no matter how much I loved this person, the relationship wasn't going anywhere. My romantic offers slowly dwindled, as did my feelings for her, and I moved my attentions to a more receptive audience. More than twenty years later, this woman, although still very attractive, is still not in an intimate relationship. She has always wanted to be single and just prefers being on her own.

When a genuine relationship exists, and one member is putting in 100 percent, he or she can be sure the relationship will succeed and prosper. As long as you give your maximum without waiting for your partner to throw in theirs, you will have a successful union. When *both* parties put in 100 percent, then the relationship will thrive and reach the greatest heights. The more one member is willing to put in, the easier it becomes for the other to do the same. If one partner holds out and the other responds by doing the same, then the relationship will be in trouble. Furthermore, giving feels best when the giver enjoys the process and is not waiting for something in return. I give my partner a massage or drive her to an appointment or give her an orgasm for the fun of doing it, because it feels good to me. She is not compelled to return the favor. When she desires to give me an orgasm or cook me a meal, she does so because she likes doing it, not because she owes me anything.

A relationship is good when both members are intent on their partners' getting what they want. Although it is nice to be loved, cherished, and cared for, it is even better to find someone whom you want to love and cherish. The best thing, however, is to find someone whom you want to love and cherish and who feels the same way about you.

〜 Happiness 〜

When a man and a woman get into a deep relationship, one that resembles marriage with or without the certificate, an unwritten contract exists between them that the man will do whatever it takes to see that the woman is happy. I know this is how I've felt with the few women I have loved deeply, and this attitude has been corroborated by our male friends and students. By contrast, I have lived with a number of women whom I was not so deeply in love with, and their unhappiness affected me to a lesser extent. The more a man loves a woman, the more her happiness or unhappiness will affect him. Women, of course, prefer their men to be happy, too. However, as we discussed in the preceding chapter, men largely base their value on their productivity, and producing a smile on the face of one's beloved and making her happy can be taken as a show of a man's productive abilities.

Our friend Robert loved to make his wife happy. When they first got together and he offered to take her out to eat, she sometimes asked him to pick the place. He loved pasta and basic Italian food, and she preferred more exotic cuisines. Whenever he chose his favorite Italian restaurant, at first she avoided telling him that she didn't want a high-carbohydrate meal. Instead, she would go to the restaurant he chose and would spend dinner being unhappy. As a consequence Robert didn't enjoy himself either. When she eventually 'fessed up and told him where she really wanted to go, and when she enjoyed her dinner there with gusto, it didn't matter to Robert that he didn't have his pasta; what mattered was that she was thrilled. When a woman is happy and having a lot of fun and her man believes he caused her joyful state, he can only respond by feeling good, too.

It can be challenging to make another person happy. Indeed, most studies we have seen indicate that each person has what might be called a "happiness quota" that remains fairly constant regardless of the circumstances. A person who is genuinely happy most of the time can be in a car accident, lose the use of their limbs, and in a few months be almost as happy as they were before the accident. At the other extreme, a person who is unhappy most of the time can win the lottery and in a short time will be as miserable as ever.

It is also apparent to us that people who are in agreement with their lives—that is, who see themselves as doing what they want to do, being with whom they want to be with, and having what they want to have—are genuinely happy. Similarly, people who are out of agreement with their lives—who aren't doing what they think they want to do, aren't with whom they think they should be with, or don't have what they believe they should have—are unhappy, miserable folk.

How, then, does one get in agreement with one's life? The next sections touch on this timeless question.

∼ Recognizing Life's Perfection ∼

Being in agreement with the way things are and wanting the things one has are the keys to being happy. This does not mean that one shouldn't have goals or aspirations. It means that the first and best step to obtaining one's goals is the realization that one's life is perfect as it is, including having specific goals and desires. Perfection as we use the word here does not mean that every hair has to be in place or that one has to have the ideal life; rather, it is the recognition that the life a person has is perfect for that person at that time and that place. When a person gets into agreement with the way things are now, the future, too, will be perfect, and whatever comes along will be more of what he or she wants.

It can be easy to say that "everything is perfect right now," yet sometimes when reality hits home, it can be difficult to put theory into action. When I was told that Vera had colon cancer and that it probably had spread to her liver, I certainly did not feel that things were perfect. I felt horrible. I fainted and actually peed in my pants. In fact, though, my reaction was a perfect response for me. Vera responded differently. She said to me and to the two friends who were with us that we would just use the experience as a reason to go higher. So you see, two people can respond differently to the same or similar experiences, and both ways can be thought of as perfect. There is no one right or perfect way.

∼ Being Out of Agreement with Life Equals Insanity ∼

When I responded with such strong "negative" emotions to the news of Vera's illness, in order to feel better I first had to get into agreement with the fact that I was feeling terrible rather than trying to resist the emotions. I had to accept where I was at that moment. Expressing emotions and giving them a name helps a person get into accord with the experience much sooner, especially if they have someone else who will listen as they process and identify the feelings. From there, a person can rearrange their value judgments to better serve them by perhaps changing their goals or attitudes. It can help to remember that being out of agreement with the way things are can be thought of as a form of insanity, if one of the definitions of insanity is a refusal or inability to face reality. Taking Vera's advice, we used the experience of her illness to go higher, which to us meant becoming more intimate and more in love than ever, and taking our friends with us on the ride.

It is also good to remember that having specific expectations and getting angry over life's failure to live up to them is quite senseless and will only lead to unhappiness. According to Alan Morinis, in *Climbing Jacob's Ladder,* the biggest sin is worry. Seen from one perspective, worry is the belief that God (or however you think of a higher power) has in store for you an undesirable, unhappy, negative life. Another component of worry is the belief that the bumps we all inevitably encounter in the road of life are unconstructive and lack any redeeming qualities or lessons. By contrast, when you trust the greater scheme of things and let go of having to control everything that happens to you, especially those events that are truly out of your control, you become more adaptable and thus more able to experience life happily. Most trials turn out to be less awful than one worries or thinks they will be. An amusing yet truthful quote from Mark Twain says, "I'm an old man and have known a great many troubles, but most of them never happened."

∼ Women Are More Comfortable with Grief ∼

What, then, can a man do to help the woman he loves be happy? First of all, he must realize that she is not going to be happy all the time. It is useful to know that women are more comfortable with a variety of emotions than men are, including grief. Most women move to grief more readily than most men. A man's response to a similar experience will often be expressed (or, more precisely, unexpressed) as apathy. When a woman is in a grief state, her partner may put himself into her shoes and assume that she must be feeling terrible, depressed, miserable, or possibly suicidal, when in actuality she may not feel too badly and may be rather comfortable in this mode. There are different levels of grief. If a man has been in a relationship with a woman for a while and can stay tuned in to her, he can tell the difference between a shallow-level state of grief she may be experiencing and a truly deep, lengthy depression.

Furthermore, he can talk to her—or better yet listen to her—and inquire about her feelings. More than once he may have to ask her questions like "What's bothering you?" "What are you feeling?" "What's got you down?" In such a case, keep asking your partner questions until she expresses herself. The simple act of showing care and concern for her will cause her to feel better. She may reply that nothing is bothering her, but if you know that something is, keep asking until she tells you exactly what's got her down. As we stated in Chapter 2, a man often wants to remedy a painful or distressing situation, but in fact the best thing he can usually do when his partner is feeling blue is just to listen and allow her to express herself without trying to fix anything. If a man can do this, he will benefit from his partner's feeling better and more loving toward him. She will appreciate that he cares how she feels. She will feel attractive because he is focusing attention on her by listening to her and allowing her to express herself. After she feels better, she will probably open up the conversation even more, thus increasing the possibility for intimacy and closeness.

As we recommended in the preceding chapter, when you're talking or listening to a woman, keep your attention on her. Resist looking around and noticing other things and people. A man gains points (or at least doesn't lose any points) when his focus and interest are only on the woman he is with. Women are more conscious, or at least more sensitive, than the average man, so a woman is going to notice when his attention wanders. She wants to know that her man will be there for her when she desires his attention. If she feels secure, she doesn't always require his attention, but she wants to know that he is willing and able to provide it when she does. At times she may be so filled up with his attention that she wants to take a break and park him somewhere for a while. (By "parking" him, we mean encouraging him to occupy his time watching a ballgame on TV, golfing, reading a book, doing chores, etc., to allow her to have some space from him.) When she is ready for more attention, she will let him know. Vera loves it when she parks me by the computer and I write her love poems. It lets her know that even though we aren't physically together, I am still thinking about her.

Although it may seem to run contrary to what we've been saying up to now, in spite of men's egos and their beliefs that they can make a woman happy by being or doing something for her, women are responsible for their own happiness. (Men are too, for that matter. More on that subject later.) In fact, this is not a paradox; it is more like a cooperative and mutually beneficial team effort. Although men can play a part in helping their women to be happy and fulfilled, happiness ultimately comes from inside a person. The more a woman is able to realize that she can choose fun and pleasure for herself over anger and bitterness, the happier she will be. The opportunity to make this choice appears over and over in every person's life, and watching for it requires a certain amount of vigilance (until with practice it becomes close to second nature). A woman who knows that men love to make her happy—or as Regena Thomashauer says in her books, "that men live to put a smile on a woman's face"—is able to express her desires openly. She knows that most men really want to know what will produce that smile, and she is willing to ask for what she wants without worrying that she will be judged negatively. She knows that a man is thrilled to hear her express her desires without holding back. She gets what she wants either because she is willing to ask for it or because she has such strong, magnetic intentions that she might as well be asking. Ms. Thomashauer recommends that women actually practice asking for what they want, since most aren't used to flexing those muscles. She suggests practicing in front of a mirror when you are alone. Practice asking for anything, whether it is having your sexual desires satisfied or getting your favorite menu item from a restaurant. A woman who is happy and who is getting her desires fulfilled becomes that much more attractive to men, who in turn want to make her even more happy. Happiness begets more happiness.

⤳ First, Love Thyself ⤳

Before a person can genuinely love and be loved by another, they must be able to love themselves. For some people this comes naturally; for those with low self-esteem it may take some time and work. Many of the exercises we've included in this book can help you increase your self-esteem. In addition, learning to love yourself can involve shifting how you look at things. Here's an example of what we mean: Almost everything we do—if not everything—we originally do for right and good reasons. Only when we look at things with hindsight does it appear that we have made bad or foolish choices. For example, maybe a person could have studied more in high school to get into that good college and get that good job, but at the time it may have seemed the better choice was to have fun and to party. However, if we knew then what we know now, we wouldn't be here to begin with. Therefore, instead of being hard on yourself for what you see as poor choices you made in the past, forgive yourself and move on. As long as you see yourself as wrong, you will continue to make wrong choices.

Thus, loving yourself is akin to approving of all the choices you have made and will make. It is closely aligned with getting into agreement with your life. It is seeing yourself as a "perfect you," rather than trying to be anyone else. It is measuring you with *yourself* as the yardstick, rather than measuring yourself against some famous model, who in reality does not even look like the airbrushed version in the magazine, or against an older brother who was a genius at mathematics while you had difficulty with the multiplication tables. The more one approves of oneself, the better one will become at whatever one tries, and the more one will be able to approve of and love someone else. You may have noticed that people who are the most critical of others are also hard on themselves. If you can't show love to yourself, how can you show it to another?

Once a person has learned self-love, the next step is often directing his or her love toward another. To learn to love and cherish someone, start by getting to know that person as well as you can. Find out about their likes and dislikes. Inquire about their goals, desires, and aspirations. Ask what they were like growing up; learn about their friends, former relationships, everything. Find out about their fantasies, both sexual and otherwise. Knowing whom you are interacting with can help you determine whether to pursue a relationship with him or her or to move on to someone more compatible. If you decide that this person is someone whom you can appreciate and love, then your early inquiries will have yielded some basic information that can help you in cherishing and caring for him or her.

Learning about another person is an ongoing endeavor. Although we've been married for over twenty-two years, Vera and I still discover new things about each other. When I think I have heard all of her stories, she will surprise me with a new one. When we were first getting to know each other, we took long walks during which we asked each other questions about our pasts and about what we wanted in the future. Today we are still taking long walks, during which we ask about each other's lives and discuss our desires and goals. Since we work as a team and enjoy similar activities, we spend much of our time together every day, yet there is always something new to share—for example, something one of us learned from talking to somebody at a party, or what we are thinking about that day, or an interesting fact I read in a book. Occasionally we pursue separate activities, as Vera likes to get manicures and pedicures, and I like hanging out in bookstores and using the hot tub and swimming pool. Afterward, we are glad to see each other even though we may have been apart for less than an hour. We treat it as a reason to hug and kiss, as if we had been separated for days. Not every couple, of course, spends so much time together. Still, no matter what your circumstances, treating each other politely, being friendly, and showing curiosity about each other will make for a stronger relationship.

∼ Taking Each Other's Side ∼

Another component of a good relationship is for the partners to take each other's side when either of them has conflicts with other people. If your partner has had an argument or disagreement with anyone, be understanding and show them you are on their side. If you think your partner can benefit from hearing another point of view, you may decide to gently share it with them later, but first let your partner know you support them and their perspective.

Even if you think your partner acted foolishly or provoked the other person, it is important to demonstrate that they can count on you to back them up. This goes especially for conflicts with in-laws and other family members. Take the side of your spouse. When people believe they have at least one other person on their side, they are usually more willing to negotiate and soften their stance. If you take the side of the party opposing your spouse, they may think the whole world is against them, which could cause them to distance from you and everyone else.

If I've clashed with someone, Vera first supports me by agreeing with me about how the other person was at fault. After a while she may bring up the idea of apologizing to the other person, so I can begin to put the episode behind me. Vera and I use the gift of apology and recommend it to our students. Whether you are right or wrong or whether you were offended or were the one who offended another, apologizing for your part in a conflict can be very helpful in maintaining a healthy psyche. Staying angry causes harm primarily to the one who is angry. Apologizing makes a person feel better by freeing them from the negative incident. Having my partner's support and understanding makes it easier for me to apologize to the other party, claim responsibility for my part in the incident or quarrel, and move on.

∾ Dealing with Conflicts and Differences of Opinion ∾

Even if a couple has a great relationship, arguments and disagreements will occur. Conflict seems to be inevitable in any close association between two people. We all have our viewpoints and behaviors, and when someone sees something differently or behaves in a contrary way, it presents some conflicts. This goes for men and women in intimate partnerships, of course, especially since the two sexes can differ in how they see things. To avoid becoming entrenched in an argument, recognize that it takes two people to disagree. This means either person can get into agreement at any time to end the dispute. Still, some conflicts between men and women will never be solved, and the couple that learns to live with their differences will be that much more functional and successful.

Here's an example: Vera is very neat and likes for everything to be in order. I am basically a messy person who tends to throw his clothes anywhere. We have learned to live with each other's idiosyncrasies in this area. I have learned to be much neater than I was when we first met, though I'm still far from obsessively neat. Vera has even learned to enjoy picking up after me when she wants everything in order; furthermore, she can get me to help her clean up by being nice and not getting upset over my behavior. On rare occasions she has even joined me in my behavior and has left the bed unmade before leaving home. Another example is deciding who wants to watch what on television. Luckily we have two TV sets, so if I want to watch a sports event and Vera wants to watch a movie, we both get to see what we want. However, when we are traveling and have only one TV, it is more fun for me to watch a movie with her than to make her watch a ball game that she cannot stand. Once she falls asleep I turn on the baseball or basketball game and watch the last inning or quarter, which is the best part of a game anyway.

So, again, although every relationship will have some conflicts, how they are handled determines whether the relationship is successful. Although at times people must negotiate with each other to solve disagreements, we do not think either party has to compromise their desires to be able do this. If one person wants to eat fish and the other wants steak, deciding to have chicken won't leave either party feeling good about it. A better choice would be to cook both foods, unless one party is willing to change their mind over what they want. I have found that when I am willing to go along with what Vera wants, whether it has to do with what we eat or anything else, she is very grateful. It also seems that when I give in and say, "Okay, let's do it your way," she becomes more willing to look at my viewpoint on the matter and consider changing her mind. On the other hand, if I resist her desires and insist that what I want is more important than what she wants, she definitely becomes more stubborn—and the chances of our going to bed and having sensual fun later diminish. It really doesn't matter which of us starts to get into agreement with the other; sometimes it is Vera who is the first to give in. Again, both parties must disagree for a fight to continue; therefore, if either party changes his or her stance of disagreement into one of agreement, then suddenly a completely new dynamic is created. It goes back to what we discussed early in the chapter about the importance of giving without keeping score. The more willing you are to give your partner whatever they want, the more willing they become to give you everything you want.

What about when the conflict is over something big, like the amount of time spent working versus being together? We have found that when a woman is in disagreement with what her partner is doing at work, she will often sabotage his endeavors. When she feels a shortage in the amount of attention she receives from him, she may create havoc and setbacks for him in his outside enterprises. Somehow things do not go smoothly; deals get changed for the worse; money problems surface—and until he changes his ways, the patterns continue. When she is in agreement with how he is dividing his attention, things miraculously become easier and seem effortless. Some women focus a lot of attention on their own outside endeavors, too, and don't seem to care what their partner is doing since they have no time for his attentions anyway. A relationship like this can go on for many years; however, we would not classify it as a great relationship but as more of an association between two parties. Of course, partnerships also exist in which both parties are able to balance rewarding outside jobs with a wonderful relationship and home life. Such an arrangement requires both partners to be very energetic and supportive of each other and of the relationship.

There is no one right way to deal with the issue of how much time to spend together. We have met many seniors who seemed to have had happy enough marriages, either while they were both working or when the husband worked. Then, after retirement, when both parties were at home all the time, they found themselves arguing more. In such a case it often works for one of the spouses to find a new job, develop a new hobby, or enlist in some volunteer work. Then the couple can go back to relating on a part-time basis, which often works better since that is what they're used to.

When a couple argues, obviously something is out of agreement between them. It is good to figure out what the issue is so it can be aired and resolved. To occasionally complain in a specific way about a specific incident is one way of getting directly at a problem, because it gives the other party information and allows them the opportunity to either make a change or take responsibility for the issue. We do not recommend a style of arguing that relies on over-generalizing—for example, using words such as *always* and *never*. Accusations, such as "You never help me" or "You always think about yourself," are challenging to respond to constructively and cause most people to react with resentment. If you're going to register a complaint with your partner, keep your comments very specific, and keep your words and your tone of voice as kind as possible. Of course, to get your partner to move in the direction you want, it is better to use positive reinforcement than it is to complain or criticize. How to do that is the overarching topic of much of this book.

Sometimes couples argue to let off some steam, and then, once tempers have subsided, make passionate love. This can happen only when both partners refrain from attacking each other with critical or contemptuous statements. It also must happen before one of the pair goes numb and tunes out the other. A fight that leads to sex can result from any issue, but it seems to occur most often when one partner is jealous over something the other did or said involving another person. People do not have to fight when they're feeling jealous, but it happens because the amount of energy generated when jealousy is involved becomes elevated to a level that most people find too uncomfortable to live with. They could have skipped all the fighting as a means of releasing the pressure and instead could have gone straight to having orgasmic pleasure, but most people are unable to start an orgasm from such a high energy level. We do not recommend getting into arguments over jealousy—or for that matter over any other particular issue—as a reliable method to get your partner into bed, but if you do find yourself in a fight, there is some hope. Remind yourself that it takes two people to keep the argument going. If one of the two gives up arguing and gets into agreement with the other, he or she can take control of the situation and possibly move them toward some sensual pleasure. On a few occasions Vera and I have made passionate love after arguing. Years later we still remember the lovemaking but have no idea what we were arguing about.

The moment doesn't even have be ruined when a couple starts arguing *while* making love, if the argument is resolved quickly and if having pleasure is more important than winning a disagreement. I recall an episode when Vera seduced me into letting her rub on my genitals by touching me sensually and pleasurably and turning me on sweetly. We started in the living room, then moved to the bedroom, got naked, and continued. Once we were naked, it felt to me as though she was just going through the motions. The original turn-on seemed to be missing, and her touches felt just so-so. I asked her what she was thinking about, and she said, "Nothing." So I told her how I felt. At first she denied that anything had changed, but then admitted that to her it seemed I did not appreciate what she was doing. I told her she did not have to continue but I would love it if she did. She said she wanted to. Once she started touching me again, I verbally acknowledged all the wonderful sensations—little and big—that I felt. This time, the sensations got better and better. We started with a disagreement and from there got into agreement, and as a result, things improved quickly. Instead, both or either of us could have continued to grow angrier, which would have been the end of that episode of pleasure. As this story illustrates, communication during lovemaking is an important way of staying conscious and remaining connected with your partner. We include some exercises for how to communicate during sex in Chapter 5.

In every relationship that either of us has been in, as well as every relationship we've heard about, couples argue about the same things over and over. Happy couples, in successful relationships, have conflicts over the same sorts of issues as unhappy ones; the difference is that partners in successful relationships are much nicer to each other about their differing viewpoints. They learn to have a sense of humor about the "predictable" responses of the other party whenever they broach the topics of contention. For example, I like to break conventional rules and minor laws, while Vera prefers to do everything by the book. Instead of getting angry at each other for being different, we enjoy our differences and the fact that we are not living with clones of ourselves. Growing up in New York City I learned to cross the street whenever possible, whether the traffic light was red or green. Vera grew up in Europe and obeyed traffic signals. We now live in California, where laws against jaywalking are enforced to some degree. By being with me, Vera sometimes gets to walk across the street when the light is still red, and she can blame me if anything bad were to happen. Sometimes we do it her way and wait for the light to change, even though no traffic is coming; this gives me an opportunity to learn patience.

We have some friends who have been together for a number of years. Their relationship is in trouble because they do not treat each other very kindly. The man often throws tantrums when he thinks his partner isn't listening to him. Predictably, however, his rages have the effect of causing her to refuse to listen to him at all. She treats him critically and tends to keep her distance from him, afraid that he might blow up at a moment's notice. Sadly, instead of growing closer as years pass, they are growing apart. It really takes two to fight and one to make up.

When a couple is arguing, either person can change the conflict by getting into agreement with the other, at least to some extent. In the case of our friends, one of them could have stepped out of their normal negative routine and gotten into agreement with the other's viewpoint. Perhaps the woman could have said, "I understand why you are angry. I provoked you into getting into this state, and I apologize for hurting you." It is very difficult to stay angry at someone who apologizes and takes responsibility for the situation. The man could have ended the conflict, too, by admitting that he was hurt before it developed into full-blown anger. He could have gotten into a dialogue with his partner, asked her some questions about her behavior toward him, and ended the conflict before it even started. Or he could have informed her that he felt hurt and angry and that he was going to take a walk until he calmed down, and then they could have talked about it sanely. Either person could have taken responsibility for the situation and avoided the pain that ensued.

There is often more than one valid viewpoint regarding an experience. If either the husband or the wife in our example had entertained this awareness, he or she could have kept his or her own viewpoint and at the same time could have understood that the other person was seeing the situation in a different context. It is helpful for people to understand that they are not their viewpoints; rather, we humans are "viewpoint holders," and we have the ability to hold more than one viewpoint on any topic or issue. Realizing this would have enabled our friends to get into agreement much more easily.

That said, some couples are just not meant to stay together, and sometimes it is in everybody's best interest to end the partnership. When the pain of being together outweighs the love and happiness of the relationship, it probably is best to separate. We will discuss anger in more detail in Chapter 4.

⌖ Who Does Make the Bed? ⌖

Up to this point this chapter has dealt mostly with shared responsibilities within a relationship. When it comes to divvying up responsibilities, a relationship works best when both partners generously give of themselves based on what they each are good at and what they each like doing. For example, Vera is much better at making the (literal) bed than I am. She is not only better at it, she cares more than I do about how it looks, and she dislikes looking at an unmade bed. I make the bed on occasion when Vera is busy with another project or is not feeling well, but in general she makes the bed probably 95 percent of the time. Although my bed-making skills are continually improving, after twenty-plus years together we've accepted the fact that they will never quite meet her standards. We are both happy with the unequal amount of labor we devote to bed-making.

As it happens, Vera's penchant for bed-making falls into a realm of activities traditionally considered a woman's domain. However, things these days aren't always so cut-and-dried. Women in the last thirty or forty years have been entering the work force in significant numbers. Before that, except perhaps during the Second World War, most women did not work outside of the home. The roles were simpler back then: Men worked and financially supported the family, and women stayed home and took care of the house and children. Since men made the money, they also paid for the dates. Women needed a man more than they do now; men were their sole source of financial support. Furthermore, fewer people (especially women) had sex before they were married; thus, couples often got married young so they could indulge.

Nowadays, with more gender equality in the workplace and other realms (e.g., the armed forces and politics) men's and women's roles are less neat and well-defined. People often have sex before marriage, so they wait longer to get hitched. Women are less dependent on men financially and sexually than their mothers and grandmothers were. The problem (if it is a problem) is that the same values on which our grandparents were judged remain in place today: Men, as discussed in the last chapter, are still largely judged on their abilities to produce and women on their abilities to attract. It is still the case that when someone meets a man, the first question they often ask him is "What do you do?" By contrast, the first question a woman often asks another woman is "Where did you get those shoes/that outfit/that haircut?"

Who, then, pays for a date if the woman earns more money than the man? A man who feels successful supposedly has a higher testosterone level than one who feels beaten, and testosterone levels affect a man's sex drive. If that is the case, how can a man win and feel successful with a woman who makes more money than he does and who wants to pay her own way? Here's the key: *A man must realize that the most important things he has to offer a woman are his attention and his willingness to serve her in whatever way he can. Money is only a "how," one tool in many that can be used to help him produce a smile on the face of his beloved.*

When Vera and I got together, I had next to no money, while she had a modest income. We both lived in a commune and had very little use for money. I didn't work outside the commune; the only income I made came from teaching an occasional course, the proceeds from which usually went to the commune. We didn't have to go on many dates, because the commune's facilities offered enough entertainment. I was, however, able to focus a lot of attention on Vera without having to spend much money, and our relationship thrived. I learned how to give her maximum pleasure, and I was fun to interact with. When we got married, I couldn't afford a wedding ring; instead, a friend had an extra ring with little gems in it, and I gave it to Vera. She was delighted with it, as she was with almost everything I did for her or gave to her. She never made me feel poor or unsuccessful. Sixteen years later, when I was able to afford an expensive ring from Tiffany's, she loved getting it as much as if it had been our wedding day. The message here for women is that a woman can make a man feel like a winner and a success—whatever he produces. When she does that, his success in producing for her will undoubtedly only improve.

(For a discussion of the practical aspects of a couple's finances, see the section "Money Matters," below.)

∽ Managing the Emotional Climate of the Relationship ∽

In general, women are better than men at relating to others. Throughout their formative years, girls are conditioned to learn relationship skills. Many still play house and play with dolls as they grow up, while many boys still play with toy guns and trucks. Whether due to nature or nurture, women are usually more in touch with their feelings and emotions, and as a result, they are better equipped to manage the emotional climate of an intimate partnership. Relationships seem to work better when both parties realize this on some level and agree that the woman is the one responsible for keeping the relationship in good shape.

Some men with big egos like to think of themselves as the ones who make the important decisions and who are "in charge of" the relationship. Most women are aware if their guy is one of these types of men. If he is, a woman might be well served by letting him believe he is the powerful one, while still skillfully managing the emotional aspects of the relationship herself. As Woody Allen put it when asked who was in charge in his relationship, he said he was because he controlled the remote control for the TV.

When both partners are totally devoted to one another and want each other to have everything they really desire, the relationship will thrive. Still, a woman's goals often reach higher than a man's, especially when it comes to the relationship itself. That's because, for the evolutionary reasons we discussed in Chapter 2, most women are naturally good at wanting things, and their goals and desires tend to promote the well-being of relationships, family, and community. It is important for a man to realize that when he supports his woman's getting her desires met, his rewards will be far greater than if he had focused solely on his own goals. This does not mean that men shouldn't have goals or that their goals are unworthy. It means only that if a man helps his partner meet her goals, he can potentially achieve great heights. A man on his own may lack confidence in his ability to meet his goals; a woman may believe more strongly in her partner's ability to produce than he does. When a man is willing and eager to fulfill his woman's desires, he receives an extra boost of energy. All of a sudden things that seemed difficult when he was alone get done more easily. The secret is that when true desire emanates from a woman, a large supply of energy accompanies it. By taking on a woman's goals and accomplishing great feats, a man gets to feel like a hero—which is one of the best feelings he can have.

We are not implying that men should work and women should stay home. This being the twenty-first century, many women now have wonderfully creative jobs. Each couple has to decide whether both partners work or whether one stays home as primary caregiver to the kids. The decision must be a mutually gratifying one that everyone feels good about. However, it is still true that a woman will value a man with a prestigious and high-paying job more than a man will value a woman with the same job.

What prevents a woman from getting her true desires fulfilled? The answer is her negative doubts about those desires. We are talking here about the same kinds of doubts that sabotage her turn-on, as described in Chapter 1. Because women are still largely valued for their attractiveness, the main doubts that surface will most likely be related to that part of who she is, just as men's doubts are mostly about their productivity. A woman who sends out mixed signals—that is, a woman who wants something but nurses doubts about her worthiness—confuses those around her who more than anything else want to fill her wishes and desires. As we've said several times, men live to deliver to women whatever they want. Men also respond to women according to the signals they receive from them. When the signals are clear, it is easy to produce for a woman and to gratify her desires. When the signals are mixed, men no longer feel as attracted to producing for her. It is like a radio that is not quite tuned in to a station: The signals are garbled, and thus either the task seems too difficult or the message is simply not understood.

It is natural for a woman to occasionally doubt her attractiveness, but the extent to which she does so depends on how worthy and deserving she feels. A little doubt won't dampen the signal too much, but a large amount will totally distort it. A man would do well to avoid increasing a woman's doubt about her attractiveness, and a woman would do well to avoid doubting a man's productivity. In each case, they are actually projecting their own self-doubt onto the other: He blames her for his own doubts about his productivity, and she blames him for her doubts about her attractiveness and her ability to get her desires fulfilled.

∼ Money Matters ∼

This part of the chapter deals with the practical side of finances. If one partner is good with numbers and the other is not, the one who is can pay the bills and balance the checkbook and figure the taxes. He or she can keep the other informed about the couple's financial state of affairs and ask for help if necessary. In our household, I manage the day-to-day finances.

Some married couples maintain joint accounts, and others keep separate accounts. As long as each party agrees with the way things are handled, continue doing what you're doing. However, if one person wants a joint account and the other believes in keeping their money separate, problems can arise. Such questions surrounding the handling of money are best addressed in the beginning of a relationship, so that both parties agree with the arrangement. Supposedly, money issues are a major cause of marital problems and divorce. We believe that marriage is a team effort, and the more the partners are willing to work as a team, the better their chances for success. Sharing at least some financial accounts promotes good teamwork. One possible arrangement is to have one joint account in addition to separate accounts for each person.

Each couple must determine for themselves whether one person will balance all the checkbooks and make all the financial decisions or whether the decisions will be made equally. Again, as long as both partners agree and stay in communication, any arrangement should be okay. Sometimes one person in a marriage, often the woman, will let the other handle all the money matters. We know a woman who let her husband manage the family finances. He often made a lot of money but at other times he got into financial troubles. He participated in some illegal deals that he was able to keep hidden from his wife for a long time. Finally his luck ran out, and his creditors began to hound him. This caused problems for the whole family. They had to move out of their home and modify the comfortable lifestyle they were used to. For another couple we know, things have worked out differently. The wife doesn't want to be bothered with the details of the family's finances, so the husband lets her know if things are flush or if things are tight, and she spends or conserves accordingly. They both seem very happy with this way of doing business, and so far everyone is winning. From these two couples' contrasting experiences, we can conclude that no single arrangement always succeeds or always goes sour. However, it also appears that maintaining open communication about financial affairs is a couple's best means of avoiding potential problems.

When two people start dating, there often comes a time when they experience some conflict over who should pay for what. If the man makes more money than the woman does, he usually has no problem paying for their dates. If the woman wants to treat occasionally, he should allow her to do so. A potentially more difficult scenario is presented when the woman makes more money than the man. In the beginning, whoever makes the offer can pay for the date. Once a couple has been going out for a while, they can discuss their respective incomes and how much each of them can afford to spend on outings. If the man isn't willing to let the woman pay his way or the woman does not want to pay for him, then they will have to be on his budget. This probably won't work for the long term; too much potential exists for conflict around money issues.

A better arrangement may be for each party to contribute to dates and vacations. They do not have to contribute an equal amount, nor even an amount that is in exact proportion to their relative incomes, but both need to be in agreement with who pays and how much. Again, as the story of Vera's and my early relationship illustrates, a man's willingness to give a woman all the attention she wants is more important than how much money he is able and willing to spend on her.

We know a woman who had dated a man for a few months when the two started talking about marriage. He was out of work and in debt, yet she insisted that he buy her an expensive diamond ring. He bought her the ring on credit, and within two weeks they broke up. She would have been better off teaching him how she liked to be pleasured than seeing how much debt he would get into for her. Her mistake was not in wanting the expensive bauble; it was that she had her priorities mixed up. Sometimes, as a testament to a woman's attractiveness, her partner may long to give her an expensive piece of jewelry and will miraculously find the money to pay for it. A gemstone is just a rock that has value because someone really appreciates it and because it symbolizes something about the relationship.

~ A Menu of Choices ~

A number of potential pitfalls can appear when a man decides to focus his energies on producing for a woman and fulfilling her desires. Women often don't express what they want; they expect men to read their minds. But men make poor mind readers. So when a man fails to act in the way his woman wants him to act or to produce exactly what she desires, she may get upset with him. On the other hand, sometimes when a woman feels safe with a man, she will express some of her desires. But a woman likes to be overwhelmed by a man's giving her more than she asked for because his doing so is a testament to her attractiveness and wonderfulness. A person cannot be overwhelmed when they receive exactly what they asked for. Therefore, most women who do tell men what they want tend to order short. They ask for something but hope that what they get will be bigger or better than what they requested. A woman does this for one of the same reasons why she avoids telling her man what she wants in the first place: She hopes that he guesses it right and thereby proves that her appetite and attractiveness are miraculously evident. Most men do not realize that most women order short. They are grateful to any woman who is able to ask for what she wants, and thus they wind up giving her exactly what she's asked for. The trouble is that she usually turns out to be less than thrilled with this response to her request, and the man is left to wonder why. So, men, it is good to know that many women order short. A woman may ask you to touch her sexually for five minutes when she really wants it for twenty minutes. She may ask for a twenty-five-inch TV set when she really would like a thirty-two-inch set.

But there's a flip side to this business. It is also important that a man avoid producing *too much more* than his woman asks for, because his doing so can cause her to be *too* overwhelmed and to feel overfull. As we touched on in Chapter 2, when a person is unable to digest all that is given to them, the excess turns to garbage. So if a woman asks for five minutes of sexual attention and her partner gives her over an hour, or if she asks for a twenty-five-inch TV and he comes home with a forty-six-inch plasma-screen set, he may be overproducing. A man who aims to fulfill a woman's desires must keep his attention focused on her reactions in order to notice if he is giving her too little or too much. He can learn from these experiences and if necessary adjust his strategy in the future.

One option is to make a woman various offers and see how she responds to them. You can create a menu of choices and observe which one turns her on the most. Do this by keeping your attention on her and also by noticing the feelings in your own body when she is responding to the choices you offer. When her face lights up with a smile and your body feels great, those are good signs that she likes a particular option. If, for example, she won't say which restaurant she wants to go to, simply list a few restaurants that you like and see what kind of a response each one gets. Then you can say, "Let's go there" to the choice that drew the best response. That way, she gets to feel like you were paying close attention to her—that you were "reading her mind." Be aware, however, that it becomes your responsibility if the experience turns out to be less than great.

The things women want—or, for that matter, the things all people want—tend to fall into certain categories. Our teacher, Dr. Vic Baranco, called them "sex, food, and baubles." Sex includes anything that has to do with attention, love, companionship, romance, and sexual stimulation. The category of food encompasses all of life's necessities, including a roof overhead, food on the table, basic clothing, and adequate transportation. Baubles include anything extra, such as jewelry, fancy cars, expensive restaurants, designer clothes, and even babies. Since anyone reading this book has the "food" category covered, we address only the sex and baubles groups here. Women want to be gratified in all three areas; however, when a woman realizes that gratification in the sex and attention category is more deeply satisfying than being delighted with baubles, she will be generally happier and more appreciative.

A man presenting a menu to a woman can make offers from more than just one category. For example, he can name restaurants that serve American, Japanese, Italian, Chinese, or French cuisine. He can also ask if she would like to be made love to before dinner, with candles, music, and the works. Maybe she would like to have dinner delivered so the romance won't be interrupted, or maybe she would like to go out after making love. Again, by keeping your attention on her while listing your menu of choices, you can easily determine her preferences.

Women, you can also present menus to men. But since the basic agreement is that men want to make women happy, know that the best way to make a man happy is for you to be happy and to cause him to feel as though he played a role in your happiness.

∼ Getting Married ∼

How do you know when it is time to take the next step and move in together or get engaged? There is no single way to tell when the moment is right. It depends on who you are, on who your partner is, and most of all on how you feel. Marriage seems to be a step in the journey of love, but it is not the be-all and end-all. Some couples are against the institution itself, and many of them have led wonderful, loving lives together. Most couples seem to make the move when it feels like the next right thing to do. Some people get married and divorced multiple times, while others, especially men, seem reluctant to do it even once. Just because two people get divorced doesn't mean they were wrong to get married in the first place.

Only in fairly recent history have people had the freedom to make their own choices about whom to marry. In most traditional societies marriages were prearranged, usually by the parents. This is still the custom in some cultures. Supposedly, prearranged marriages have the same likelihood of success as ones in which the spouses choose each other. In our society men most often make the actual marriage proposal. Still, the woman has a lot to do with whether her partner even considers the possibility. Sometimes questions and comments from a man's friend about his plans for marriage trigger him to begin thinking about the matter and planning his proposal. In some ways proposing marriage is just like any other seduction, in that a person has a goal and a plan to persuade someone to do something that hopefully will be pleasurable for both parties. In other ways it is not like a seduction because marriage must be discussed and planned for by two individuals.

When a man wants to propose marriage he does not always know in advance how his partner will respond. Though her response is important, questions about how she will respond must not sway him from actually making the proposal. Asking someone to marry you is a significant way to expose your desires and feelings toward the person. They could say no to you, in which case you will have to step up your seduction and the amount of loving attention you show them to get them to say yes, but if you do not take the risk and ask, then the answer will be no for sure. It is also okay to ask more than once. At least you will have opened the door and shown your lover how much you feel toward them. Only ask when you feel ready to do so, but do not let the possibility of rejection sway you from asking.

Some people think they should have a certain amount of money before they get married; for others this isn't even a consideration. Just because you cannot afford a ring or you have little money it doesn't automatically mean you should put off getting married, and just because you have more than enough money it doesn't necessarily mean you should get married. Nor does the fact that a person has limited financial resources always mean that he should refrain from buying an expensive ring for his beloved. Again, all of these issues depend on the people involved. A man will be able to produce for a woman who shows genuine appetite, and if she really wants and enjoys a ring and it means a lot to her, then he will find the ring easy to come by and to pay for.

We have a few more thoughts on the topic of engagement rings. On their own, diamonds and other jewels are simply shiny, colorful rocks, just as furs are simply the skins from dead animals and expensive wines are simply fermented fruit. What gives these things life is the person who wears the jewels or furs or who imbibes the wine. No matter what size the rock, it is the woman who gives a ring value when she values and appreciates it. When a diamond ring becomes more important than the person giving it or when the size of the stone is more important than the love between two people, it is probably a bad omen. The fancy ring I gave Vera after we'd been married for several years looks beautiful on her finger not merely because it is an exquisite piece of jewelry, but mostly because it symbolizes the preciousness of the love we share.

Every society has traditions surrounding the wedding ceremony. Weddings can be beautiful, but many times both the preparations for the festivities and the event itself end up being more stressful than they are pleasurable. Putting together any large social gathering is not easy. Add to this the fact that weddings carry much more significance than any other celebration, and you have a recipe for potential anxiety and nervousness. The bride, often together with her mother, is the one primarily responsible for planning a wedding. The groom can earn some points by helping where he is wanted and by otherwise not demanding lots of needy attention.

∼ Babies and Children ∼

Some women seem to lose interest in sex for a couple of years after giving birth. For others, the opposite can be true. After Vera gave birth her libido actually increased. Especially if a new mother experiences a decrease in sexual desire, it is important for her partner to continue being a friend and to continue making her pleasurable offers, but to do so without acting demanding and needy. This is a great time for men to hone their masturbation skills so they can release sexual tensions regularly.

For a child's healthy emotional development, both parents need to be involved in the child-rearing. The mother is usually (but not always) in charge of the care and nurturing of the infant, but it is important that the father contribute as much as he can to the child's emotional growth and physical care. He can also make sure that his partner is well taken care of. Finally, parents who have children of all ages would do well to arrange for a baby-sitter on a regular basis in order to allow them some time alone together to unwind, communicate about adult topics, and possibly enjoy some physical pleasures.

∼ When Your Partner Is Sick ∼

When a woman is ill, her partner often feels that somehow he is to blame. Because of the unwritten contract that says a man will do whatever it takes to ensure that his partner is happy, a man usually feels responsible for his partner's well-being. This means any illness she suffers may very well cause him to feel bad, too. I know I feel terrible whenever Vera gets sick. I would almost prefer to be sick instead of her, because then I would have more control over the situation. I feel almost impotent about my inability to make things better for her. My worry probably puts pressure on her that makes it more difficult for her to recover. Such an attitude doesn't necessarily make a man a better nurturer or caregiver. In fact, it may actually cause him to be more irritable and less appealing to have around.

Partners often have different levels of ability and willingness to act as caregiver when the other is ill. This was very much the case for one couple we knew. Whenever the husband was ill or even had a checkup, the wife accompanied him to the doctor. She scheduled his appointments and made sure he got to them on time. By contrast, whenever she had to see a doctor, her husband did not want to go with her. She either went alone or, if she wanted some support, asked a girlfriend to go. The two were fine with this arrangement. In particular, the wife was glad that her husband wasn't with her at the doctor's office because he was irritable whenever she was sick.

∾ Flirtations and Affairs ∾

From a discussion of partners' roles in various everyday scenarios we move now to the sensitive topic of outside affairs. This section doesn't cover every aspect of the subject, just certain ones that we believe are important to comment on.

Any discussion of affairs has to start with the topic of flirting. Flirting is fun. It is important to realize that when two people are in love, it doesn't mean they have to give up flirting with others. Getting mad at one's partner for being flirtatious with members of the opposite sex will make the partnership weaker rather than stronger. A relationship works best if both parties are allowed to enjoy themselves as much as they can without too many strings attached. That said, however, going to bed with someone other than your partner is a boundary that may be best to keep in place.

In a few cases it can work for partners to have lovers in addition to their primary one, but a lot of thorough communication and work are required to pull it off so that everyone wins. In most cases such a scenario is too sticky to execute appropriately. Our society and conditioning tell us that having outside lovers is such a negative transgression against the primary relationship that a couple must either be very evolved and do it openly, or simply not care about each other or the consequences.

Vera and I once lived in an experimental commune where it was okay for people to have more than one lover. The key was that everything was above-board; that is, there were no secrets. Some women who were very sexually gratified arranged for their partners to have specific lovers of the woman's choosing. In these cases the woman did not mind sharing her man with her girlfriends because she felt totally taken care of by him. This scenario functioned better than in cases where the man did his own choosing. Women who wanted to could also have affairs. The openness around it all was very effective in helping everyone involved to feel okay about it. The conditions were very controlled and had been agreed to by everyone. To pull off the same in the absence of similar circumstances would be much more difficult.

Outside of that type of arrangement, we have known only a few women who had serious relationships with more than one man at a time, and in each case the relationships dissolved after a while. A man who has successful, open relationships with two or more women at a time occasionally is successful in his various relationships, but they are usually problematic and difficult. As the character Lazarus Long states in Robert Heinlein's novel *Time Enough for Love,* the Chinese ideogram for the word *trouble* is two women under the same roof. The only way it can work well is if the two women genuinely like each other and stay in communication. One benefit of this type of threesome is that the two women can get extra turn-on from each other.

If one has a secretive affair and one cares about their primary relationship, the best thing to do is to come clean with their partner. Otherwise, the transgressor will find himself or herself growing to dislike his or her partner, who, in turn, will sense the transgressor's dishonesty. People whose partners have had illicit affairs are often more angry about having been lied to than about the actual transgression.

The main reason why women in our society have affairs is because they don't receive enough attention from their partners. A woman may have a beautiful home and lots of nice stuff, but perhaps her man is away a lot, causing her to feel lonely and neglected. A woman who is in a situation like this can grow so angry at her man that she is a prime candidate for starting an affair with the proverbial milkman or mailman—or whoever shows her some attention and care. Women, if you find yourself feeling neglected because of your partner's lack of attention, it is important to have a heart-to-heart talk with him as soon as you recognize what's going on. If you wait too long, it will become more and more difficult to communicate with him. If you never tell him otherwise, he may think you are perfectly happy. Tell him you appreciate your lifestyle but that you would prefer to be with him more than the things you are surrounded with. Let him know what you really want. If you have to go to a marriage counselor or take a course or workshop together on improving your relationship, then do it.

Men may balk at going to a counselor or enrolling in a marital-improvement course. They may think they are being punished or are losing if they must go outside the marriage for help. (It's the same story as when men resist having to stop and ask for directions while driving.) Yet it is good for men to know that marital-improvement workshops can be very enlightening and beneficial, even if you have a sound relationship. Likewise, think of going to a marriage counselor as getting help from a coach who knows what he or she is doing.

Women, how can you persuade your partner to get help for the relationship if he resists doing so? First, as we said above, if the relationship is on the rocks and you are unhappy because of a lack of attention from him, sit him down for some serious talking as soon as possible. If you've been feeling this way for a while and have failed to address it with him, take responsibility for not having brought it up before now. In as nice a way as possible, let him know how you feel and what you want. Ask him for some ideas and input about how the two of you can arrange to spend more pleasurable time together. If and when you decide you want to see a counselor or talk to a relationship coach or enroll in a workshop or read a book together, tell your partner what you want. Have confidence that he will say yes. Do not have any doubts about whether or not he will agree. Do not ask him if he would like to do it; that would give him too much wiggle room. Make sure he knows how important this is to you if the relationship is going to survive. A lot of men will avoid counseling unless they think their marriage is on the line. However, don't make threats you are unprepared to carry out. Don't tell him you'll move out or kick him out unless you mean it. If your partner complains that you have stopped making love with him and says this is why he has become more distant from you, honestly ask yourself whether that may be true. Remember (and this is true for everyone), if you want to be loved, you have to be lovable; if you want to be adored, you have to be adorable; and if you want attention you have to be fun.

～ Sexual Satisfaction ～

The final topic we'll touch upon in this discussion of intimate partners' roles and responsibilities is sexual pleasure. We'll say it again because it bears repeating: We believe it is important for men to be willing to give their partners all the attention they desire—including sexual attention. Through all our years of teaching sensual techniques, we have worked with scores of students. We have observed that many, if not most, women have barely scratched the surface of the sensual pleasure that is available to them, while most men lack any clue about how to produce this pleasure for women. We recommend that women learn the art of having wonderful orgasms and that man learn the art of producing them for women. Most men know how to have an orgasm, and most women know how to give a man an orgasm. The reverse is often not the case, but it can be learned, by both parties. Again, a key part of the formula is attention: When a man puts 100 percent of his attention on his woman's pleasure, she can experience what it feels like to be sexually gratified.

It may take some time for a woman to fully develop the ability to feel intense pleasure and have great orgasms. While she's learning, her man must have patience and must let go of expectations of receiving much sexual attention from her in return until she has been sexually filled up. Then, once a woman is sexually gratified, she develops into a better lover herself. She can take her man to sensual places he has never been before. This is one of the reasons why we place a lot of importance on the woman's sexual satisfaction. A woman who experiences intense pleasure every time she and her man go to bed will be way more willing to say yes to his invitations or even to make requests of her own. By contrast, when she harbors doubt about her ability to have orgasms and to feel much pleasure, there is very little motivation for her to want to have a sexual experience. The same is true for a man; that is, if he feels impotent, there is little reason for him to want to go to bed and to "fail" again. The difference is that most men are not impotent—they are able to get erections and have orgasms—whereas most women don't have orgasms every time they go to bed, and when they do, the orgasm is often not very intense or extended. A man who knows how to stimulate a woman's genitals with his hands (one of the main techniques we teach) will never be impotent—at least with regard to his ability to please her orgasmically.

When a woman first learns of her natural ability to feel intense pleasure, as we fully describe in our two books on extended massive orgasm (see Bibliography), she is eager to have many dates in bed so she can learn to feel even more. This is an opportunity for her man to explore her new aptitude with her. It is a chance for him to become a hero in bed, something that most men only dream of. As we stated above, once a woman discovers the wonderful pleasure that is available to her, she may at first want to focus all the couple's attention on it, seemingly to the exclusion of giving her man an equal number of orgasms. This state of affairs will only last so long; after a while she will resume wanting to give her man pleasure. A man would do well to grant her these desires; they present him with an incredible opportunity to be a hero. Furthermore, her own education in receiving sensual pleasure will make her more proficient in producing it for her man. Once both parties understand this, there will be no shortage of orgasms for anyone.

As if all these reasons weren't enough, a sexually gratified woman is much more fun to live with. Sexual satisfaction allows a woman to open up in other areas of her life that she may previously have been afraid to explore.

Whereas most people are used to the kind of lovemaking in which the partners pleasure each other simultaneously, another emphasis of our teaching is for partners to learn how to pleasure each other one at a time. We do not ask our students to stop doing the former, only to add the latter to their repertoire as another enjoyable activity. We have found that the pleasure to be had from an orgasm produced by this one-at-a-time method is the most intense that is humanly possible. This is because when both parties concentrate on one person's pleasure or orgasm, it is easier to really focus their attention and to communicate effectively. The person being touched gets to just lie there and feel the sensations without having to exert any effort or energy on pleasuring their partner. Likewise, the person doing the touching has that specific job only, which precludes their worrying about whether or not they are being equally satisfied or touched properly.

∽ The Importance of the Clitoris ∽

So what is the trick to consistently bringing a woman to these heights of pleasure? Stated in short, it's all about the clitoris.

The clitoris is such an amazing organ and of such vital importance to a woman's sexual pleasure that it is astounding how little has been written about it or verbally passed down through the ages. I had attended medical school for two years and been married for five before I heard the word *clitoris* at age twenty-five. Fortunately, in the past few decades more information has become available about the clitoris, but there is still way too little information available in relation to this organ's significance.

The only function of the clitoris is pleasure, which cannot be said for any other part of the human body. Again, this is because in anatomy as in other realms, men are the norm against which everything else is judged. For centuries the vagina has been thought of as the receptacle for the penis and therefore as more important than the clitoris. Little girls are informed about their vaginas and are sometimes even taught to call their entire genital area "vagina" (or another, less sexual, made-up word, like "mumu"). Freud wrongly taught that women had two kinds of orgasm: the clitoral orgasm, which he referred to as "immature" (although at least he knew about the clitoris), and the vaginal orgasm, which he described as the "mature," or more deeply felt one. In fact, women have only one kind of orgasm and it is clitorally based, whether or not the clitoris is being directly touched.

Even today, years after the so-called sexual revolution, we find that more than a few women still do not know the exact location of their clitoris. Of the ones who are familiar with the clitoris, a large percentage still feel inadequate because they are unable to regularly reach orgasm during sexual intercourse. This is the main reason why so many women fake orgasms when having intercourse: They don't want to appear "abnormal," and they don't want to offend their lovers by causing them to worry that they (their lovers) are unskilled at lovemaking.

The fact that a man might think of himself as a poor lover if his partner is unable to have an orgasm during penile penetration shows how little men know about the clitoris and its huge involvement with a woman's orgasm. We find that most men these days have at least heard of the clitoris, which is better than when I was growing up, in the sixties. Yet even if they've heard of it, many men still don't have a clue about where it is, how to expose it, how to touch it, and how important it is to a woman's pleasure. If this describes you, fear not. In Chapter 7 we offer detailed techniques for how to stimulate a woman's clitoris.

In our research we have found that the head of the clitoris, as its most sensitive part, is the best place to touch it for maximum pleasure. It also feels good to stimulate the shaft of the clitoris and the G-spot, which is the location inside the vagina where the roots of the clitoral nerves end. Although women usually find it very pleasurable to have their G-spot stroked, it is less sensitive than the head of the clitoris. It is best to stroke the G-spot while simultaneously stimulating the head of the clitoris. We also include more information about pleasuring the G-spot in Chapter 7.

Women really love to have their clitorises touched, although sometimes when a woman has never been touched there skillfully, it may take some time and practice getting her clitoris to feel as good as it can. (We describe how to deal with this issue in Chapters 7 and 8.) We think it is extremely important for a woman to masturbate and explore her clitoris and all of her genital area if she is going to have a great sex life. This is exceptionally important when she is first starting to learn about her sensual self. For both sexes, it is always good to have the ability to pleasure yourself sensually, although once you have trained your partner thoroughly, he or she will be able to take you even higher than you can take yourself.

Over the years, many of our female students have said that they cannot get off with a guy but can reach orgasm when they masturbate. This is because they have been unwilling to teach and show a man how they like to be touched on the clitoris. Some of them expect to get off via intercourse and when it doesn't happen, they are quick to blame the man. A man holds some responsibility if he has failed to take the time and make the effort to learn how to pleasure a woman. Many men still believe that a woman should reach orgasm through penile penetration, because that is the way men have orgasms easily. It only takes one member of a couple to realize and communicate to the other that the way to give a woman optimum pleasure is by involving her clitoris.

~

Our introduction to the topic of sexual satisfaction may inspire a couple to explore more reasons for going to bed together. The next chapter continues this discussion and also points out how anger can dampen the flames of sexual desire.

✧ EXERCISE 3A ✧
Anonymous Good Deeds

This exercise asks you to do something nice for someone—either someone you know or a complete stranger. (Some people call these random acts of kindness; however, if you do them regularly, they won't be so random.) The best way to do these good deeds is to do them anonymously. By doing a good deed for someone without his or her knowing that you did it, you will be doing it only because it feels good to give, rather than because you expect something back from the person. This is a very powerful exercise. Doing it will make you feel good and cause you to like yourself more, and it will open you up to creating a better, more fulfilling life for yourself.

Guidelines and pointers: Good deeds can be anything that makes someone else's life better and that you enjoy doing. You don't have to spend any money, or you can if you want to. You can secretly clean up the yard or sidewalk in front of someone's home. You can send a person flowers with an unsigned note saying, "The world loves you." You can pay someone's bridge toll. Think up your own good deeds, and, remember, keep them anonymous. Watch the movies *The Magnificent Obsession* and *Pay It Forward* for a greater perspective on this exercise.

✧ EXERCISE 3B ✧
Revealing Inner Feelings

This exercise offers an opportunity for couples to become more intimate. It works best if both parties are willing to show the other more about who they are and if both agree to refrain from jumping on the other or finding them wrong for revealing who they are. The two partners sit facing each other (rather than on the phone or in a car). One person asks the other to reveal something they have not revealed before. The second person answers with whatever comes to mind, without worrying about whether they in fact have never before revealed it or about how significant it is. After the respondent finishes, the questioner says, "Thank you," and asks the same question again. Do this for five minutes; then questioner and respondent reverse roles. Or, if you are getting something out of a particular line of discussion, you can stay with the original roles for longer than five minutes before switching.

∽ *Chapter Highlights*

- ◆ If partners in an intimate relationship keep score of who did what for whom and how much and who owes more, the relationship is doomed.

- ◆ Giving works best when the giver does so because he or she enjoys it rather than because he or she is waiting for something in return.

- ◆ The first and best step to obtaining one's goals is the realization that one's life is perfect as it is, including having goals and desires.

- ◆ Learning about another person is an ongoing endeavor.

- A component of a good relationship is for the partners to take each other's side whenever either of them has conflicts with others.

- It is important for a man to realize that when he supports his partner's goals and desires, his rewards will usually be far greater than if he is focused solely on his own goals.

- A woman likes to be overwhelmed by a man's giving her something that is bigger and better than she asked for, because his doing so is a testament to her attractiveness and wonderfulness.

- A man wanting to produce for a woman who doesn't readily express her desires can make her various offers and see how she responds to them. He can create a menu of choices and observe which ones turn her on the most.

- A sexually gratified woman is more fun to live with. Sexual satisfaction allows a woman to open up in other areas of her life that she may previously have been afraid to explore.

- When it comes to satisfying a woman sexually, it's all about the clitoris.

CHAPTER 4

You are the out to my in.

The cause of that grin.

The way to my path,

The reason I laugh.

Getting Ready for Bed

Overcoming Resistance to Pleasure

*W*e are the products of countless generations of humans (and before that of generations of our primate ancestors—and so on, all the way back to the earliest multi-cell life forms) who had successful sexual experiences. It is in our genes to want to have sex, to desire to be touched and to be pleasured by another person. This is true for both males and females. Why, then, does it often seem so hard for a man to convince a woman to go to bed with him, even if the two are married or in a committed relationship? Some women, of course, are sexually aggressive or "hot to trot," but that seems to be the exception to the rule. This chapter explores this phenomenon as well as other forms resistance can take, including the problem of anger as a hindrance to sensual pleasure. It also offers ideas for overcoming these barriers.

◦ The "In-and-Out" Fallacy, or Why Many Women Resist Sex ◦

An answer to the question of why women in general are more resistant to sex than men has to start with a discussion of sexual intercourse. It makes sense that females must be choosier about when and where to engage in sexual intercourse since they are the ones who bear most of the burden in the outcome of any sex act that produces offspring. However, not every sex act between a man and a woman produces a child, humans being one of the few animals that can have sex at any time during the female's reproductive cycle. In addition, a variety of safe contraceptives exist that were unavailable to our ancestors.

In fact, intercourse is different for women than it is for men. The vaginal wall has no pressure-receptor nerves; which means the pleasure available to women through intercourse is negligible. Some statistics indicate that about 70 to 80 percent of women *do not* experience orgasm during intercourse, whereas almost all men do. It makes sense, then, that women would resist doing something that not only carries the risk of pregnancy but also isn't even much fun. Furthermore, intercourse in our society has typically been associated with the missionary position, with the man on top, which implies the woman's submission. (The words *missionary* and *submission* even come from the same Latin root word: *mittere*, "to send.") There are dozens, if not hundreds, of different positions for intercourse, so to do it the same way every time, especially in the missionary position, is a perversion. As Dr. Vic Baranco wrote in the magazine *Aquarius,* "As a sweaty, hairy beast rutting for its own gratification, the man imprisons the woman, pinning her like prey to be devoured beneath his obsessive, hormonally driven thrusting. Plowed into a mattress or a pile of pillows, having only the air produced by the two bodies to breathe, enveloped in his alien smell, and entrapped in the forest of his heavy body and limbs, ceasing only at his will, she feels degraded, defiled, and used without her consent."

Dr. Baranco's description may be an exaggeration of our human sexual condition, but it does provocatively illustrate why intercourse is usually inadequate to bring women to the wondrous heights of pleasure that many men assume it does. This is the "in-and-out" fallacy we refer to in the heading of this section: Many people, both men and women, erroneously believe that women do—or at least should—receive tremendous pleasure from the "in-and-out" action of sexual intercourse—just because men do. It is another example of men's experience being the gauge by which all human experience is measured.

As we stated in the last chapter, the key to maximizing a woman's sexual pleasure is stimulating her clitoris. Some women either have developed specific techniques to stimulate their clitoris during penetration or are lucky enough to be built so that the clitoris is close to the introitus (the entrance to the vagina). However, in most women the clitoris lies too far away from the vaginal opening to be easily stimulated by the penis's thrusting action during intercourse. (Little research has been done on orgasms in other animals, but in most female mammals the clitoris seems to lie closer to the vaginal opening than it does in humans.)

There are some exceptions to the general rule that women are less eager than men to engage in intercourse: Once or maybe twice a month, during the heat cycle, many women do have sexual urges that include a desire for penetration. For most men, however, doing it only once a month is not enough. Therefore, a man must learn to make sex more fun for his partner than it is has been for her in the past, and this means he must take pleasure from learning how to stimulate her clitoris with his hands and mouth. In her book *Sexual Selections* Marlene Zuk quotes psychologist Carol Wade as saying, "Sex is not a soccer game. The use of hands is permitted." A woman who has been stimulated to orgasm before insertion will enjoy penile penetration much more than if she had received no prior clitoral stimulation. Some people call this foreplay, but we think the term is misleading because there is nothing "fore-" about it. In fact, clitoral stimulation is the height of pleasure for a woman.

Vera and I have dedicated our lives to teaching people how to give and receive fantastic orgasms. Most of our study and research has focused on the practice of stimulating a woman's genitals, specifically the clitoris, with one's hands. Yet to this day when most people think of sex they connect it with intercourse. The word *manual* or *oral* has to be added to the word *sex* to denote what would otherwise signify intercourse. According to the prevailing viewpoint, if intercourse isn't involved, then it isn't real sex. Supposedly some young women even think of themselves as virgins until they have had missionary-style sex. In reality, however, there is simply no way that a penis can pleasure a clitoris nearly as wonderfully as a person can do with the hands and fingers or even with the mouth. Specific guidelines for doing so are provided in later chapters.

It is worth repeating that a woman who experiences wonderful pleasure every time she goes to bed is more likely to want to go to bed, while one who is sexually frustrated will show less desire. Therefore, the man who learns how to pleasure a woman with his hands will have a huge advantage over men who are still playing soccer in bed.

∽ Teach Your Children Well ∽

From generation to generation, either through genetic transference or perhaps through communication from their elders, girls appear to be taught to resist their urges and desires to have sex until it is with the right person at the right time in the right place—and even then to still resist giving in easily. As we pointed out above, women's resistance to sexual activity makes sense not only because women carry the entire burden of bearing children and most of the burden of rearing them, with all the implicit repercussions on their bodies and lifestyles, but also because sexual intercourse is inherently less pleasurable for women than it is for men.

In our present era, with the sexual revolution behind us and with information on clitoral stimulation and female pleasure readily available, will mothers take their daughters aside and teach them about this wonderful organ and its capabilities? Will mothers tell their daughters that the head of the clitoris has about eight thousand nerve endings, resulting in more concentrated sensation than the most sensitive part of the penis yields? Will they tell them that the clitoris is the most sensitive part of the human body, male or female, and also the only organ whose sole function is that of pleasure? Will parents tell their male children about the clitoris? About how to pleasure girls without the worry of pregnancy or the spread of disease?

We think it would be great if folks were more informed as youngsters about how to pleasure one another without the so-called risks that come with uninformed sex. The right age at which a young person should first be given this knowledge depends, of course, on his or her physical, mental, and emotional maturity levels. We do not expect a major, immediate shift in how people educate kids about sex, as our culture is not one that is based on pleasure, but hopefully what we propose here will eventually take hold and become part of young people's basic training about sex and sensuality. Meanwhile, we're glad that in general our society is more advanced in this knowledge than it was in past generations, and that at least people can find good information in books and on the Internet.

❧ Issues from the Past ❧

Other issues besides a woman's reluctance can get in the way of a couple's enjoyment of sensual pleasures. Sometimes these problems can benefit from professional therapy. We occasionally refer clients to a therapist. Whether a person seems to need therapy and will benefit from it usually depends on how much responsibility he or she has taken for his or her past experiences and current situations. The more someone is aware of their own responsibility for their life decisions and the more they choose to benefit from that awareness, the faster they are able to transform their life into how they want it to be. When a person seems stuck in blaming the past for their current situation, we recommend that they go to a specialist.

We have known many people who endured some form of molestation when they were children. We have also known a few people who believed they had suffered childhood abuse when in fact it turned out that they either had imagined it or were persuaded by a therapist's suggestions. We have known couples who've had problems in the bedroom and difficulty becoming more intimate because one of them—usually the woman, but sometimes the man— was sexually abused as a child. Each person responds differently to the experience of childhood abuse. Some must go through years of psychotherapy to gain control of their lives, and some use the experience to create a better life for themselves without utilizing therapy as an aid. Individuals who have a history of childhood molestation and who want to move beyond it must either get into some kind of agreement with their past, realizing that they are adults now and that their partner loves them, or seek professional help. Some people go to therapy for a while and then experience a flash of meaningful insight, an epiphany of sorts that helps them move on by giving them a new perspective. For others, attaining a transformative outlook seems to be an ongoing process. We have known people who benefited greatly from going to therapy and having someone regularly listen to them, and we have known others who seemed to get nowhere with therapy. Discussing negative past experiences with an intimate partner can sometime help a person to get on with life, and at other times a person is best served by finding a good therapist to help them realize their true power and potential, thus freeing them from having to live as a victim of the past.

We have noticed that people often like to hold on to their problems, for whatever reasons. Maybe past difficulties were the most interesting and exciting things that have happened to them. Even though the charge on an incident is negative, they regard it as an important part of their lives and thus are unwilling to resolve it and move beyond it. Or maybe they feel righteous about their anger and somehow enjoy being the victim, therefore refusing to forgive those who transgressed against them. The spring-cleaning exercise located at the end of this chapter can help you to rid your psyche of negatively charged past events.

We have had some students who, when they were given new and more exciting challenges, such as learning to have and give extended massive orgasms, were able to let go of their negative past experiences and move on. There is only so much room in our psyches for awareness and excitement. Taking on new challenges can potentially engage the part of a person's mind that previously was occupied by old problems.

～ The Problem with Anger ～

Men, you have a choice about how to feel if your woman seems resistant to going to bed. You can be out of agreement with the situation, or you can use it to learn to be deeply grateful for the differences between men and women. (We'll talk more about this later in the chapter.) As we stated earlier, when we find ourselves out of agreement with the way things are, it creates unhappiness because we believe we are losing. By contrast, when we are in agreement with our circumstances, we are winning. Men hate to lose, and when they lose, they often become angry—in this case, angry toward women or at least toward their partner. They think women should be as eager as men are to go to bed, and when this expectation or perceived right is violated many men get angry.

Anger is an obstacle to most if not all goals. In order to obtain a goal—the goal under discussion here being to enjoy sensual pleasure with a woman—a person has to see clearly. Anger fogs a person's view and negatively affects his or her attention. To complicate matters, women are very sensitive to other people's anger, and they often believe they have more reasons to be angry than men have. Therefore, an angry man is very unattractive to almost any woman.

Entire books have been written about why women feel they have the right to be angry, but the topic is worth exploring briefly here. Since the rise of agricultural society, and maybe even before that, women have been regarded in almost all cultures as second-class citizens. As we pointed out earlier, to be the second-class citizen when there are only two categories (in this case the two sexes) makes women lower-class citizens in relation to men. Men are considered best; women are considered worse. Women have been getting the short end of the stick for thousands of years, and the main tool they've had for improving their lives was to use their "pussy" as a means of viable exchange. Even though nowadays women are treated more equally under the law and have other ways to improve their lives, they are still angry over the millennia of inequality they've endured. It is just another reason to resist sex with men.

Our teacher, Dr. Vic Baranco, used to say that people get angry when they perceive that a right has been violated. Believing that one of our rights has been violated is another way of finding ourselves out of agreement with things. Women know they are at least as smart as (if not smarter than) men, just as valuable to society as men, and just as good as men. Yet they are regarded as worse than men. This violation of what women see as their natural right to be treated and regarded equally, particularly in this age of increased information and communication, can make them livid. Then, when a man gets mad at a woman, he reminds her of her own anger, and the result is usually an escalation of angry, ill-considered behavior on both sides.

Dr. Baranco also believed that people have no rights to begin with, and that thinking we do is the big mistake that gets all of us into trouble. One of our favorite characters is Lazarus Long in Robert Heinlein's book, *Time Enough for Love*. Lazarus has lived for thousands of years and has compiled many sayings and truisms. One of them is that people have no rights; they have opportunities, but no rights. If people have no rights, then they have no reason to become angry. We agree with this line of thinking. We believe that humans have opportunities and choices to make, but we have no innate, "God-given," natural rights.

If a driver gets angry when someone cuts him off on the freeway, it means he believes he has a right to drive without anyone's getting in his way. I get mad when I have to wait in line in a store, as if I had a right to go straight to the cashier. In this country we have something called a Bill of Rights; we are told we have the right to life, liberty, and the pursuit of happiness. But think about it. We do not actually have a right to live. We are fortunate to live, grateful maybe, privileged perhaps, but we do not have a right to live. Someone can run us over, shoot us, or bomb us—and what then does the "right" do for us? It is the same with liberty. We have liberty until someone takes it away from us. Rights don't really do anything for us, except perhaps trap us into feeling pain if we perceive that they've been violated. We do not go around whistling and singing because we are so happy to have the right to vote. But should someone take away this perceived right and prevent you from voting, you would become irate and unhappy. A better perspective would be to feel privileged to have the opportunity to vote (or to live, or to be free). This way, you get to feel good most of the time.

When people hear this concept for the first time, they often argue with us. Sometimes they get angry over the notion that they do not have any rights. Our editor even suggested that we refine our argument to distinguish between "cosmic" rights and "political" rights. Whether rights are defined as cosmic or political, we believe that human beings do not have any whatsoever. We know this may be difficult to grasp at first, but if one is willing to look at each right individually, one will realize it is actually not an innate right. It is at best only a temporary privilege. One man got really upset when we suggested that he had no rights. He insisted he had the right to breathe. Later that day he got some food stuck in his windpipe; someone used the Heimlich maneuver to save his life. Afterward, he called to tell us we were "right"; he did not even have the right to breathe.

Noticing that you are angry may be the first clue that one of your boundaries has been violated. In this case, anger perhaps serves some useful purpose. It is, however, possible to notice that your boundaries are being violated before you reach the point of anger or at least before your anger becomes full-blown. To do so, one has to be alert to one's feelings and be aware of the fact that some perceived right has been violated. Before feeling anger a person usually feels other emotions, such as feeling hurt or debased. Responding to these emotions by saying "Ouch" or "That hurts" may in some instances be enough to ward off the anger. We are not saying it is possible for most humans to avoid anger all the time, but it is possible to lessen its duration and intensity.

Perhaps anger has served as a springboard for creating social and political change in areas such as civil and feminist causes. Still, consciously noticing that an injustice is occurring without letting it affect one's ability to reason calmly is a more effective tactic than demonstrating angrily. And we do have a choice about whether or not to act angrily. The show of anger is quite selective. If a small, unarmed person were to attempt to violate one of my rights, I would act differently than if the same right were violated by a large, armed individual. That is to say I would get mad if I thought I could get away with it, but if someone had a gun pointed at my head, I would be on my best behavior.

∼ Anger or Orgasm? ∼

Anger mimics sexual excitement and orgasm in most of its physical manifestations. Just as sexual excitement does, anger causes increased heart rate, increased breathing, flushing of the skin, and increased perspiration. The only way in which anger does not mimic sexual turn-on is that there is no wet pussy or hard penis.

It is so easy to get angry. It costs nothing going in. All you have to do is find some right you feel has been violated, which is simple for most people. It is expensive, however, after the fact. Chronic or habitual anger is very destructive to the body. It causes damage to the circulatory system, especially the heart. It is probably one of the major causes of heart disease and other ailments, right up there with smoking cigarettes.

By contrast, even though sexual turn-on and orgasmic bliss exhibit physical manifestations similar to anger, they are totally its opposite in other ways. They cost energy and intention up front. You have to find a partner, come up with a reason to do it, and focus deliberate attention on the goal of experiencing pleasure. Furthermore, sexual pleasure is beneficial to the body, causing it to produce powerful endorphins that create feelings of well-being. Positive sensual attention makes a person appear and actually become healthier. After a good orgasm the skin glows and the face looks at least ten years younger. Women use makeup because it mimics what they look like when they are turned on and orgasmic.

So, if one has a habit of choosing anger over pleasure, how can one change that pattern? To offer insight into this question we will first touch on some of the ways in which the two sexes differ in how they "do" anger. In general, women are much more covert about their anger than most men are. They do not usually go around throwing things and putting their fists through doors. They keep their anger close to them so that often the men living with them have no idea they have so much wrath locked up inside. The trouble with a woman's hidden anger, besides the fact that it causes the man to lose, which is usually the reason why she does it this way, is that in denying pleasure to her partner she is also denying pleasure to herself. It is a double-edged sword, and it cuts her as much as it does him. When a person yells and screams and acts overtly angry, afterward they often feel bad about having behaved intolerably, so they become remorseful and try to be more loving and kind. By contrast, a person who fails to express their anger but rather keeps holding on to it continues to function under its negative influence. The best thing to do is to realize that one does not have any rights; then the anger will disappear. The fastest way to stop being angry is to just stop being angry as soon as you realize that you are. Of course, this is easier to say than do for many folks. Some people are helped by attending anger-management groups, reading self-help books (I liked *Climbing Jacob's Ladder)*, or participating in individual therapy.

Climbing Jacob's Ladder offers a technique to help with chronic episodes of anger. It suggests that a person keep a rubber band in their pocket, and as soon as they notice that they are beginning to feel the slightest amount of anger that they should place the rubber band on their wrist. This is a conscious act that serves as a trigger for the person to realize what they are doing and to ask themselves what they really want to accomplish. We have some friends who were too easily angered and obviously were hurting themselves and their relationships with their ugly behavior. We told them about the rubber-band trick, and they tried it. It seemed to create an opportunity for them to notice and be more conscious of their bad habit and to respond more calmly and pleasantly to everyday aggravations, whether being stuck in traffic or waiting in a slow supermarket line.

A woman who wants to do something about her anger will benefit by noticing when she believes that her rights have been stepped on and by paying attention when someone, especially her partner, says or does something to negatively stimulate her. She will be best served if she expresses her feelings to the other person as soon as possible. She can tell him what he said or did that caused her to feel hurt or as though she were losing. If captured and expressed quickly enough, these negative feelings can be discharged without turning into full-fledged anger with all of its repercussions.

A great way to reduce anger in general is to put more of one's attention on creating fun and pleasure and to choose the most pleasurable route when one comes to a fork in the road. A person has only so much space available in their head at one time. There seems to be room enough for one emotion and only a few thoughts. When we fill our heads with pleasure and with pleasurable thoughts, there is no room for anger, and it will go somewhere else, where it is more wanted.

◅ The Pursuit of Pleasure ▻

So although we may not have a true bill of rights, we do have the possibility to pursue happiness, and that is our best option. Actually, we think of it less as a pursuit and more as a decision to choose pleasure whenever possible, to observe life as it is, and to be in agreement with it. If you adopt this mindset, happiness will pursue you. As we put it in a previous chapter, a woman who is happy attracts good things to her, things which create even more happiness. It is the same as the principle that says the rich get richer, but the currency is joy rather than money. The same goes for men. For example, a man can choose to be thrilled with the fact that women are different from him. He can rejoice that women do not want to have sex with every man at any time and at any place. He can create a game out of these differences, and if he learns how to play it well, he will benefit much more than he had originally hoped. Learning to appreciate the differences between the sexes also increases the value of the goal of experiencing sensual pleasure with a particular woman. The greater the obstacles to achieving a goal, the greater the worth and importance of the achievement of the goal. If a woman were to say yes to you every time you wanted to have sex, after a while (maybe not at first) you would feel that it was too easy, that there was no real game involved. The value of the prize would decrease.

One game men and women can play is to surrender to pleasure with each other. We are not talking here about a physical wrestling match (though that can be fun, too), but rather about a game in which a person feels safe enough to actually desire the pleasures offered by the partner. However, when a person is angry, there is no way he or she will choose pleasure or choose to surrender their nervous system to another. They have to be able to give up their anger at least temporarily if they are going to engage in a loving, sensual experience. The more anger a person holds on to, the less they will be able to surrender to the possibility of fun. We believe that if one is going to pursue pleasure, it is best to pursue it with all of one's capabilities and gusto. Anger cuts into that gusto and prevents a person from experiencing sensual possibilities.

When a woman is pissed off at her lover for slighting her or ignoring her—or for whatever reason—she will be unable to allow him to succeed by creating fun for her and giving her orgasmic pleasure. She will refuse to surrender her nervous system because it is filled with negative currents. She may pretend to surrender and may pretend to give him pleasure, but a man who is conscious and feeling will immediately be able to tell that something is up. By contrast, a man who is unaware or is mostly into himself will fail to notice her lack of enthusiasm, which provides further reason for her to be enraged at him.

A person who is willing to suspend their anger—we call it leaving it outside the bedroom door—can always pick it up on the way out. No one is going to steal it while you are in the bedroom having fun. A funny thing about having pleasure is that it fills a person with so many wonderful feelings that afterward most people will most likely forget to pick up the anger waiting outside the door. When someone experiences a great orgasm, he or she feels good and looks better for hours afterward. These people usually wear a hint of a smile, if not a full smile. They are nicer to everyone for the rest of the day. The world looks brighter, the person involved is more generous, and he or she has little use for anger.

Pleasurable feelings last for a while after the pleasurable experience, depending on the circumstances a person gets involved with and the kinds of attitudes and outlooks they are exposed to. After enough negative stimulation, it is only a matter of time before most people lose the positive edge they got from the pleasurable event and revert to feeling more negative toward life and those around them. A person who is somewhat aware and conscious can notice the negative bombardment coming their way from everyday events and can somehow either get into agreement with it or escape to a place or create a situation that offers more pleasure.

To surrender one's nervous system, one has to trust that the person they are surrendering with (notice we did not say "surrender to," as the surrender is actually to one's own greater pleasure) knows what he or she is doing and isn't going to cause any physical, emotional, or mental harm. To surrender is to make oneself very vulnerable, therefore doing so can be a challenge, especially the first few times. This is why it is so important for men to learn about women's bodies and about how to give women pleasure and to know what kinds of things are good to say and what kinds of things are better left unsaid.

Many women surrender their nervous systems only partially. The better a man is at focusing his attention on his partner and at playing with her resistances, the sooner she will give up control, most likely bit by bit. There is no need to rush to total surrender. Getting there takes time and can be part of the game. As long as it keeps getting better, you can know that you are going in the direction of pleasure.

∾ Overcoming Resistances ∾

Even I, who, I might boast, knows more about women's orgasms and pleasure than most—if not all—men, know that Vera isn't going to say yes to every sensual offer I make to her. This actually makes it more fun, as there would be no game if every time I said "green" she said "go." Women are not like traffic lights, or like men. But they like to receive offers because it validates their attractiveness, so it is very important to continue to make requests for sensual fun, even when your partner doesn't say yes every time. Women like to have pleasure and to receive orgasms; a woman wants the man to take that extra step to show that he is willing to do whatever is necessary to seduce her. Plus, as we've said, a man appreciates a goal that much more when he has made some effort and overcome some obstacles to obtain it. Each resistance a woman offers is a chance to advance one's seductive abilities.

There is a Russian saying that when a diplomat says yes it means maybe, and when a diplomat says maybe it means no, and when a woman says no she means maybe, and when a woman says maybe she means yes. Sometimes a woman says no and there is no way in hell a man can change her mind. At other times she says no and a little more work will convince her to say yes. A man has to understand the difference between the two kinds of no's. Even when the no is the inflexible kind, more play and seduction may cause her to consent to some pleasure in the future. Sometimes a woman will say yes and get the man all engorged, and then she will change her mind and say no. A man has to respect this change, and the quicker he does the more willing she will be to say yes again.

As you can see, the game of overcoming resistances is itself about making love. Do not look at each rejection as a rejection of you, but rather as a temporary rejection of an offer that if properly or differently made could have a different outcome. Know that women have been conditioned to say no, that nice girls are not supposed to want to do that, but in actuality they are usually just looking for the right excuse to have more fun. There are no exact formulas, and no one is ever sure how much effort will be required to turn a no into a yes. Make the overcoming of her resistances part of the sensual act or experience. That is, have fun every step of the way. Use your seductive skills to get her to admit that she wants pleasure and a fun time. Women sell (and men buy) all kinds of excuses to avoid having fun. For example, "Not now, I have a headache," "I'm too full," "I'm too tired," "I'm not in the mood," "We'll wake the kids," or any of the other millions of pretexts. I don't think there is a school or a class where women go to learn all these excuses, but we've compared notes with other couples, and they all report similar lines that cause men to fold and give up.

One seductive trick is for a man to actually think up new reasons why the woman should not join him for a fun, pleasurable time, and then quickly reverse the reasoning to show why it is a good idea after all. A friend of ours told his wife that he would love to make love to her but that they couldn't, as they would be late for work. He had earlier put their clock ahead forty minutes, so when he told her they actually had forty extra minutes, she went for it. This trick would probably work only once. Play with various strategies and have fun with the game until you have her at a point where you can make your move and she will go for it. The game-playing shows her that you are willing to make the extra effort to be more intimate. It shows that you are paying lots of attention to her and will continue to do so for however long it takes. A fun strategy is to bring the woman to a place of saying yes and then continue with the seduction until she has to beg you to touch her. (Note that this tactic is *not* recommended for beginners who are new at the seduction game. A woman wants to surrender but will resist doing so until she feels safe enough to do so. A man who is unsure of his seductive skills can come off as tentative, which will prevent her from surrendering to him. If he is trying to get her to beg him and she doesn't go that route, then the whole experience can quickly go downhill.)

Everything being equal, it makes sense that a person would say yes to pleasure and no to pain. However, everything is not equal, and as we have made clear, there are all kinds of excuses a person can use to avoid choosing pleasure. It is far easier to say no to pain than to say yes to pleasure. Saying no to pain is easy because the energy is right there, pushing you away. With pleasure you have to devote energy to making it happen, and many people are just too lazy to do so, even though the reward for choosing pleasure far exceeds any energy spent initially creating it. In making a bid for pleasure it is also important that one be knowledgeable and confident in one's sexual abilities.

It can be helpful to come up with creative ideas that will gently push your beloved toward choosing pleasure. Make the most of opportunities presented by birthdays or anniversaries or the giving of gifts to go to a nice hotel for one or more nights. There are countless other ideas you can exploit in the name of fun and pleasure; you just have to look for them. We know a couple who like to go to a hotel near where they live. They hire a baby-sitter and deliberately plan a day and a night of fun in bed together. They enjoy themselves so much that they do this at least six times a year. The hotel represents pleasure to them. It acts as an aphrodisiac even though the woman's desire is ultimately responsible for the success of the outing.

∽ Monkey See, Monkey Do ∽

Many people do things because everybody else is doing them, a fact that presents opportunities both for enjoyment and good and for pain and sorrow. Pagans used to have holidays when the normal rigid rules of behavior were replaced with fun, frolic, and sexual escapades. Because everyone in the village was doing it, women allowed themselves to openly express their more instinctual sexual appetites. In the late 1960s and early 1970s a larger percentage of the population was into "free" sex. Because so many people were doing it, it became the trend. When Vera and I lived in a community that explored sex and sensuality, the norm was for women to express their sensual desires. We had classes with rules that said the participants had to have an orgasm every day or maybe three or more times a day. In one class the participants had to give and receive a three-hour orgasm once a week. Because it was in the structured environment of a sensuality course, women felt free to choose pleasure over the usual prudery that our society generally promotes. Under these circumstances it was the proper thing to do to express desire and ask for pleasure. Both the women and the men were generally gratified and happy. However, as soon as the course was over, there was a huge decline in the number of orgasms and pleasurable experiences people had, until the next class started.

When people are newly falling in love they do not seem to need as many excuses or reasons to get into bed. A natural chemistry supplies the energy and the fuel for pleasure. As teachers, Vera and I see our role as helping our students go from a good place to an even better one. It would seem to make sense, then, that our work would be excellent for couples who are newly in love and are already having sensual fun together. However, when things are going well, people believe there's no need to fix anything, and most folks seem to think that getting sex instruction means you're trying to fix something. Therefore, most of our students are either couples who have been together for a while or single people looking for a partner. When we do get a newly in-love couple, we are able to give them excellent ideas to enhance what great fun they are already having, as well as some helpful tools they can use for the rest of their lives when the chemistry does lessen.

∾ Drugs ∾

How do drugs and alcohol affect the sensual experience, including the overcoming of resistance? If a man has drunk a lot of alcohol, his penis may not get hard or may stay erect longer than a woman has interest in it. This is known as "whisky dick" or "whiskey hard-on." Other circumstances and other substances, including drugs such as Viagra, can have a similar effect of modifying the female's control of the erection. This happens because alcohol functions to inhibit the amount of pleasurable sensation a person can feel. It may not anesthetize a person to the degree that ether does, but it was used for that purpose at one time. A small amount of alcohol may loosen up some people's inhibitions; if they want to, they can drink the equivalent of one glass of wine before stimulation without its adversely affecting the sensual experience. However, loosening up with alcohol is unnecessary if the people involved are already open-minded, eager, confident, and willing to have a sensual experience.

Marijuana can have a similar effect of loosening up the inhibitions without dulling the senses. Some people report that it actually sharpens the senses, but this may or may not be the case. Again, only a small amount is necessary to decrease inhibition. However, many people have weird mental side effects, like paranoia, from marijuana. If you do, the drug will not help you to surrender in bed. We aren't too familiar with the designer drugs such as Ecstasy, but it seems that many of them can cause quite rapid damage to the brain even if taken just a few times. We knew people who used to take LSD to enhance their sexual encounters. We still believe the best way to feel it is to do it without any drugs at all.

～

In order to go to bed and have pleasure you can see the importance of knowing how to seduce your partner to go there in the first place, and then of knowing your way around his or her genitals. We will present more techniques in the next few chapters, but for a much more detailed exploration of the topic we also recommend reading our two books on extended massive orgasm (*Extended Massive Orgasm* and *The Illustrated Guide to Extended Massive Orgasm*). Although the titles may seem intimidating, they are all about pleasure and how to have more of it, whatever your level of sexual ability. You should also now understand the significance of anger as the enemy of pleasure and the difference between sex and soccer.

✧ EXERCISE 4A ✧
Spring Cleaning

This is a very valuable exercise and one you can do as often as necessary. It seems the more resistant a person is to doing this exercise, the more they could benefit from it. Our minds are not refrigerators, and therefore the thoughts we hold onto that carry an emotional charge will begin to decay in a short time. It is best to stay up-to-date in our communications with others, thereby keeping our minds clean and ready for the next event. Most people fail to do this, however; instead, they hold onto thoughts for too long without expressing them. This exercise allows you to clean your mind of emotional garbage, thus preparing you to communicate more productively with others.

You can do this exercise with a friend or even with a tape recorder. It is best _not_ to do the exercise with your intimate partner if the emotionally charged stuff is about him or her. If you want to do a spring cleaning about someone else, for example your parents or boss, then it is okay to do it with your spouse.

If you do the exercise with another person, whom we will call the "monitor," he or she sits opposite you and makes eye contact. The two of you can sit on chairs or on the floor. Don't do the exercise over the phone or in a moving car. The monitor starts the session by saying, "Tell me something you want to clean up," or, "Tell me something you want to clean up about Cathy." You then respond by articulating whatever emotion or thought comes up, even if it is not specifically about "Cathy"—just whatever first pops into your mind. The more specific the description, the better; that is, if you talk about an event, name the specific place and time of its occurrence. So, instead of saying, "I am so pissed at Cathy because she always finds me wrong," it is better to say, "I am pissed at Cathy because yesterday afternoon while we were in the restaurant having lunch she made fun of me because in her opinion I did not leave a big enough tip." The monitor then says, "Thank you," and repeats the question. Continue until you feel better and cleaner. You can also mention things that carry a positive emotional charge, such as something you _like_ that someone did. Again, the more specific the description, the more valuable the exercise.

If you do the exercise talking into a tape recorder, ask yourself the prompting question, give your answer, and then say thank you.

Sometimes the same answer will keep coming into your head each time the question is asked. This is okay, as it may take talking about it a number of times before the charge is dissipated and you feel clean. Keep repeating the same answer if that is what comes up for you.

The purpose of the exercise is to free your mind of clutter and negative emotions. The purpose at this point is *not* to figure out how to communicate about the issues related to the person involved. It is important that the monitor understands this and doesn't repeat what you say to anyone. Choose only a monitor whom you can trust to keep what you say private. At the same time, it is also true that after doing the exercise enough times you will be better able to communicate with the person you had the emotional charge about. For example, if the subject is your boss, after doing a spring cleaning about what's bothering you, you will be better able to approach your boss and communicate to him or her without an emotional charge interfering with what you say.

If you prefer, you can write down your answers to the question and then destroy the document, or you can tape over the recording. However, the exercise seems most effective when done with a monitor. Just make sure he or she is trustworthy.

✧ EXERCISE 4B ✧
Imagining Desires Fulfilled

People often say, "If I only had more money, life would be better" or "If I only had a girlfriend, I would be happy." In fact, to be happier you do not have to actually get from point A to point B; you just have to imagine that you are already at B.

Spend a few minutes each day imagining that your heart's deepest desires have been fulfilled. Allow yourself to experience the feelings and emotions that result from these dreams coming true. Visualize that things have turned out just like you want them to. Pretend that whatever has to be accomplished for you to feel good has already happened. All these steps can make you feel happier. And remember that feeling happy acts like a magnet for more happiness.

Even the simple act of smiling can make you feel better. Our brains are huge and creative, and by being more optimistic and positive you will not only be happier, you will also get more of what you desire.

❧ *Chapter Highlights*

♦ Women's resistance to sexual activity is understandable not only because they carry the entire burden of bearing children and most of the burden of rearing them, with all the implicit repercussions on their bodies and lifestyles, but also because sexual intercourse is inherently less pleasurable for women than it is for men.

♦ We have opportunities and we have choices to make, but we have no innate rights.

♦ We have a choice about how and when we display anger. If a small, unarmed person were to attempt to violate one of my rights I would act differently than if the same rights were violated by a large, armed individual.

♦ A person cannot possibly surrender to pleasure when they are filled with anger.

♦ The game of overcoming resistances is itself about making love.

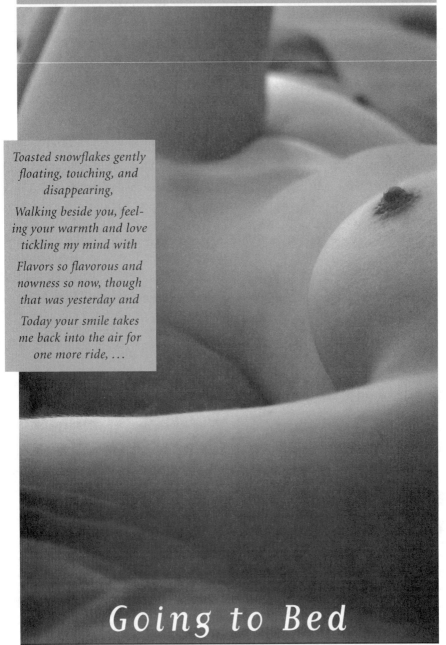

CHAPTER 5

*Toasted snowflakes gently
floating, touching, and
disappearing,*

*Walking beside you, feel-
ing your warmth and love
tickling my mind with*

*Flavors so flavorous and
nowness so now, though
that was yesterday and*

*Today your smile takes
me back into the air for
one more ride, ...*

Going to Bed
Sensuality and Integrity
for Sexual Pleasure

... One more peak lasting

*For however long lasting lasts, quivering my
soul, if I have one, to the beat of your*

*Heart, to the rhythm of your swing, to the
harmony that you bring to life, knowing just*

*When to stop, oh just one more peak as we
lay in each other's arms, legs intertwined like
two vines*

*Seeding the earth with dreams of lovers
found together by the morning sun,*

Peaking one more time,

*Through the window of your wisdom and
your willingness to bring the*

*Best out of me and anyone else. So glad,
so very glad to have you
in and out and around and over and under
and anywhere*

you happen to want to be. I am yours for

One more peak.

*I*n this chapter we begin exploring sensual activity. We discuss the importance of being in the moment, expressing
your feelings, and demonstrating integrity. We also offer a
radically revised definition of orgasm. Finally, we describe the possibilities of
using fantasy to enrich an already fun sex life.

Remember that we use the bed as a metaphor for any place where two (or
more) people can enjoy sensual pleasure with one another, It doesn't have to
happen in bed; it can be on the floor, in the back of a car, in the woods, or anywhere else. And the sensual pleasure we talk about can involve anything from
kissing you partner to touching his or her body from head to foot (including
and excluding genitals) to oral or coital sex. People can enjoy an almost infinite

number of sensual activities in an almost infinite number of places. That means there is no excuse for being bored in bed.

Even if you do something similar to what you've done before, no two sensual experiences are exactly alike. Each one will be different based on who you are at the time, how you are feeling, and how your partner is feeling and being. Sometimes you might kiss your partner only on the lips; at other times you might cover his or her face, neck, hair, ears, and cheeks with kisses, or explore the inside of his or her mouth with your tongue. We have included exercises at the end of the chapter to enable you to explore your partner's body and find out how and where he or she likes to be touched.

∼ Be Here Now ∼

There are two important things to keep in mind to help you create as much pleasure as possible during a sensual experience. First, when you kiss or touch someone, do it in such a way as to pleasure your own mouth or hand rather than to produce a particular effect in the other person. That is, even if you're the toucher (as opposed to the one being touched), take as much gratification as you can from the act itself. Second, stay focused in the present moment. Place as much of your attention as possible on the current experience. Enjoy and take delight in the act you're engaged in, without letting your mind wander and without wondering what is going to happen next. If you do find your mind wandering, don't beat up on yourself or feel like a failure. Simply bring your attention back to the present moment and to the sensations you're feeling. You may need to do this several times during an episode of lovemaking. That's okay. Just do it again … and again—as often as necessary. With practice, you'll find that it takes less work to stay present.

Making love in this way allows you to stay focused on the pleasure at hand and thus to get the most out of the experience. Enjoy the sensations with all of your senses: Smell and taste your partner's unique essence; tune in to his or her voice and bodily sounds; notice the beauty and signs of arousal in both of you; be fully aware of the touch of each deliberate stroke. You can also use your sixth sense, or conceptual thought, to fantasize, if doing so enhances your experience. (We talk more about this at the end of the chapter.)

∾ Starting from Flat ∾

Two people can start a sexual experience from any number of emotional states. Sometimes both parties are extremely turned on and experience something like animal heat. They seem unable to keep their hands off each other. This is the so-called sexual chemistry that people talk about. It may be the easiest point from which to begin to have sex, but to depend on it can be detrimental, as there is no way to determine how long you'll have to wait for it. Between new lovers this ecstatic state may last up to two years but is usually shorter. Once a couple has been together for a while this magical chemistry often fails to materialize.

Two people can also begin a sexual experience by simply deciding that they want to. To pretend to be in the throes of some sexually chemical intoxication if you don't actually feel it is counterproductive to the sensual journey. Human beings are one of the few species that can have sex at any time of the month or year, irrespective of the female's reproductive cycle. This means humans don't need to feel something akin to "animal heat" to enjoy a successful and gratifying sensual experience. The truth usually, if not always, sets one free—sexually and otherwise—so to start with a falsity will only cause a person to get stuck later. The best thing two people who are not feeling terribly turned on but who nonetheless would like to make love can do is to express where they are emotionally. We call this admitting that you're feeling flat. Being flat is not a bad place. In fact, it is a higher or more positive state than feeling angry, lousy, or like you're losing at something. It does, however, take some energy to start from flat.

Once a couple agrees they are feeling flat, they have taken the most difficult step and often by then will be in positive emotional territory. From there, once they begin the sensual ride, there is no telling how high they will go and how many ecstatic sensations they will encounter. There is no difference in the amount of pleasure that can be experienced or in the orgasmic potential that can be reached if you start from a state of "animal heat" versus starting from flat. Between feeling flat and feeling "hot to trot" are all the levels in between, and any of them is an excellent departure point for fun and pleasure, as long as one is truthful about where one is coming from.

At the other end of the spectrum, when a person is in a negative emotional space, it is best for the couple to talk more, with the intention of getting to flat or good, before going for better and higher. It is not difficult to create a flat emotional state from a negative one. Feeling negative is like having "bad" chase you, and it is easier to run from "bad" than it is to run when things are no longer bad. To go from good to better is a challenge, yet it is probably the most fulfilling path possible.

∼ Deliberate Pleasure ∼

We believe it is an excellent idea for people to deliberately plan for pleasure. It is important to create a specific place and time to enjoy sensuality. If a person waits for the "pleasure fairy" to come to their rescue, it may be a long wait. The pleasure fairy is much more likely to visit you unexpectedly if you regularly invite her in. You can do so by arranging your life to allow for delightful, fun experiences. Then the pleasure fairy will know where you live and will be able to find you more easily.

One way to plan for pleasure is to talk with your partner about what constitutes an ideal sensual experience for you and, perhaps even more important, for your partner. This way when you orchestrate an event, you can create it in precisely the way your partner likes it. You can plan what you will do, for how long, where, and with what accoutrements. When asked what they would like as part of a private pleasure party, many people resist providing straight answers, possibly because they feel vulnerable about exposing their sensual desires. Men, if this is the case with your lover, as discussed in Chapter 3, you can present her with a list of ideas and then watch the response on her face to see which ones bring a sparkle to her eyes and which fall flat.

Here are some examples of sensual menu items you could present to your beloved. (Women who want to seduce their partners can follow the same general suggestions.) You can ask her if she would like to start by receiving a back rub or if she would like to have her legs or any other part of her body lightly touched. Or perhaps she wants to have her genitals stroked from the get-go? You can ask what position she would like for the two of you to be in when you stroke her clitoris. Would she like to be in a sitting position or lying side by side? (We recommend our book *The Illustrated Guide to Extended Massive Orgasm* for descriptions of several hand-to-genital positions.) You can offer to "go down" on her or ask if she wants to "go down" on you. Perhaps she would like to be spanked or tied up, or maybe she wants to tie you up. You can also offer different positions for intercourse.

The possibilities and the ways you can offer them are limitless. You do not have to present a complete menu or even a partial one every time you have sex, but the ability to do so appropriately and at the right time will prove to be a welcome and worthwhile addition to your bag of tricks. When presenting your menu, remember to keep your attention focused on your beloved to see how she responds to the various offers. This is where paying some extended massive attention to her is useful. Also be aware of any stirrings in your own genitals, as this is a sign that she is intrigued by one or more of your ideas.

If you have been with the same partner for a long time, you probably know what sexual activities he or she likes and dislikes. Still, it is a good idea from time to time to discuss each of your preferences and perhaps to introduce some new ideas into the mix, perhaps by looking at books about lovemaking and pleasure. Couples who have been together for years often follow the same routine each time they make love. This is not in and of itself a bad thing, but it can lead to a couple's doing things on remote and thereby feeling less than is possible. Introducing new elements into your love life will help to spice up something that is already good. And if your sex life isn't that great to begin with, reading about new perspectives and learning some fresh techniques may just make it great.

Once you're in bed with your partner, things may or may not go according to plan. No matter what happens, be grateful that you are together and have scheduled some time for fun. You are not tied to any single plan; there is room for change and adventure and new vistas. It is way more important to have fun than it is to stick to some regimen just because you think you should. You may just want to lie there and hold each other at first, with or without any genital touching. Or maybe one or both of you had a bad day. You may need to spend time dealing with problems that arise and seem to block your plans. Often such obstacles are just the means by which people resist pleasure. It is frequently possible to dismiss them by promising to take care of them later. You will be surprised at how many problems will have miraculously disappeared once "later" arrives. Some issues may require your attention, but if a person is dedicated to creating fun and delight, he or she can find a way to make pleasure the priority and to quickly dispose of whatever may come up to hinder it. Resistances to pleasure are very common in our puritanical society. They almost definitely show up occasionally in one form or another. Take care of them as necessary while realizing what they are: nothing more than our conditioning making a last-ditch effort to stop the fun. The more you can enjoy resistances and have fun playing with them, the less power they hold over you and your partner.

∼ Doing It in Exotic Locations ∼

Consider experiencing pleasure with your partner in new and exotic places. Being creative in where you have sex increases your ability to feel more. If you always have sex in the bedroom, enhance your love life by sometimes doing it in other rooms. Making love on a soft rug on the living room floor in front of the fireplace, if you have one, can be very romantic. I once had a girlfriend who loved to enjoy sensual experiences outdoors. I planned lots of hikes to remote areas so we could spread the sleeping bag out on a grassy knoll or in a pine forest and play with each other's bodies. An occasional romp in the woods can be very fun and can also spike up the playfulness when you're back in familiar surroundings at home. Remember the excitement of doing it in the backseat of a car when you were young? Think about "going parking" with your lover in a remote, scenic spot. Or play with each other under the table in a fancy restaurant. These sorts of encounters are erotic and thrilling because doing them involves breaking some minor social taboos. Plus, they cause you to find a new appreciation for the wonderful comforts of home and bed the next time you plan a fun date there.

Going to almost any hotel or vacation spot tends to increase a couple's pleasure quotient. It seems that every time Vera and I spend the night away from home we also spend more time than usual in each other's arms. In our everyday life we are together pretty much all the time, and we enjoy a wonderful and regular love life, but when we go away, whether for one or two nights or for one or two weeks, we are even more sexual. It's not that we have more time to make love (although for many couples this may be true); it's that being in new and unfamiliar surroundings adds to our libido.

When you spend creative energy coming up with new places in which to enjoy sensual experiences, your partner will see your willingness to have more fun with him or her and will appreciate you for it—which in turn will increase the likelihood of your enjoying even more sensual dates together. This is especially true if the target of your desire is a woman. Women really do want to have fun; therefore, a man who is open to more ideas about how to create delightful experiences will have more fun with the women in his life.

∼ Integrity ∼

An important topic to address in any extended discussion of sensuality is that of integrity. It is crucial for a man to demonstrate integrity in deciding whether to engage in certain acts. Zorba the Greek said it is a sin for a man to refuse a woman's offer to go to bed; however, once in bed he must do only what feels pleasurable and avoid doing things simply because he thinks he should or because he feels obliged to. Specifically, this means that if a woman says she wants to have intercourse or perform fellatio or do any other sexual act, but the man senses that in fact she doesn't really want to, he must resist until he has talked with her more and his feelings about the situation change. By talking and asking questions he can find out what is on her mind and what her true desires are. As we have discussed, women crave attention and sometimes will say things or do things or ask for things to prove to themselves that they are desirable and worthy. So although she says she wants to have sex, what she really may want is your attention and your willingness to focus on her exclusively. She may want to be admired and found sexy and may think she has to have sex with a man to achieve this. In this situation a man has to go with his gut feelings and tell the truth in a nice way about what he senses. This is a part of making love. It is not only touching another's flesh but also seeing the whole person. It is true intimacy (or "into me see"). A woman appreciates a man who demonstrates this kind of integrity, although she may at first act miffed. She will feel safe trusting him with her real feelings, which in turn will cause her to surrender more fully once they do go to bed.

The woman's integrity is also important to the outcome of the shared experience. The difference is that although a man may do and say things to a woman to convince her to perform certain acts, he cannot make her body respond in any specific way. She creates her own turn-on; she is its ultimate source. She therefore must do only what she really wants to do, and if the man seduces her or convinces her to do something she thought she didn't want to do, in most cases she will be empowered by taking responsibility for being in agreement with the act, rather than feeling victimized by it. However, as we said in Chapter 1, we do not condone seduction and manipulation that lead to a person's doing something they later regret or that cause anyone harm. Gray areas exist between consensual and nonconsensual acts wherein a woman (especially a young woman) can be talked or coerced into doing something she later regrets. We know of a woman who had to deal with infertility issues arising from an STD she contracted from having unprotected sex when she was in her twenties. When she reviewed the situation years later, she understood that she had lacked good boundaries back then. At the same time, she also realized that the man she was with had taken advantage of that lack of boundaries by "talking her into" having sex without a condom. Both awarenesses were empowering for her. There's a fine balance here, and that is why it is so important for both parties to exercise integrity and consciousness. (This woman's story also provides another example of why it is important to teach our adolescents about the pitfalls and consequences of coitus and the benefits and advantages of manually induced pleasures.)

So the man says yes or no depending on how he feels in response to the woman, and the woman says yes or no depending on what she wants and desires. A man can say he wants to have intercourse, but unless his penis is erect there is little he can do about it. A woman can say she wants to have intercourse, and again unless the man's penis is erect there is little he can do about it, but if she really has the appetite for intercourse, his penis will become engorged in a heartbeat.

Sometimes a woman will say she wants intercourse when what she really wants is more loving attention paid to her body, for example for her clitoris to be touched and stimulated. A man who is sure of himself will point this out to her nicely. He can tell her he would love to have intercourse but at this time it feels like it would be more appropriate to play with her genitals. A man who lacks the confidence to say this sort of thing may instead think there is something wrong with him for being unable to "get it up." He may decide to end the sensual interlude entirely or may become angry and abusive to the woman because he thinks she is torturing or ridiculing him.

∼ Now that You're in Bed, What Next? ∼

We pointed out in the last chapter that intercourse isn't the be-all and end-all of sexual experiences, especially for most women. What else, then, might constitute a sensual encounter?

Vera and I often begin our lovemaking by kissing, hugging, cuddling, and talking. After a while, we usually include some genital contact, during which we take turns being the toucher and the touch recipient. Probably 95 percent of the time, I touch and stroke Vera's body before she touches and strokes mine. Every now and then Vera will stroke my body first, but very rarely. Sometimes I stimulate her to intense orgasm and she returns the favor by rubbing on my body afterward. At other times after her orgasm we have intercourse. Touching Vera and producing wonderful sensations in her body is often enough to satisfy me, so occasionally we end our lovemaking after I bring her to orgasm. If afterward I still desire being stimulated and she does not feel like stroking me, I have the option of rubbing myself.

Occasionally Vera has said that she wanted to have intercourse with me when in fact it did not feel like the time was right, specifically because my penis was flaccid. I might answer by saying something like, "With what?" which makes her laugh. When I continue to rub on her and take her higher, I can feel sensation building in my loins. Once it feels right, I'll tell her that if she still wants to have intercourse I am now ready. She usually takes me up on the offer.

If intercourse seems to be on the menu, be aware that it is just as important to bring a woman's genitals to engorgement and readiness before intercourse as it is to engorge a man's penis. When a woman is sexually stimulated, her entire genital area, including the clitoris (see Figure 5.1), fills with blood. The more she is stroked the more the area becomes engorged (up to a point). The clitoris usually starts off very small, hiding under its hood, but once it is

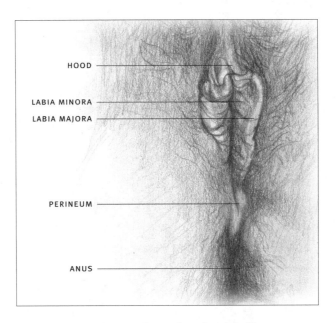

FIGURE 5.1. Outer female genitalia
showing the hood covering the clitoris

touched properly it can become bulbous, enlarged, and totally exposed (see Figure 5.2). In addition, as blood fills the genitals they change color to a deeper red, pink, or purple. A woman appreciates it if you notice the changes that occur in her body as she grows more excited and inform her of what you see and feel.

Sex can be experienced with a sense of wonder and thrill and also with a sense of humor. One doesn't always have to take oneself so seriously during lovemaking. Sex is supposed to be fun, but when a person's sense of self-worth is attached to his or her sexual abilities, the mood can turn dark and depressing if the person is still rather unskilled in bed. When people base the success of a sexual encounter on whether or not the man's penis gets hard or either party has an orgasm, sensuality is lost. Being sensual is a moment-to-moment experience involving a person's total attention on what is happening right now—not what might happen in five minutes, such as the big bang that most people associate with the end of the sex act (male ejaculation). When one's attention is somewhere other than the present moment, one fails to feel all of

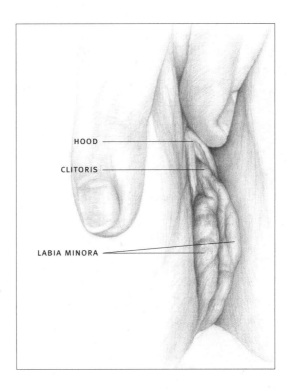

FIGURE 5.2. Pulling back the hood with thumb (right) to expose the clitoris

HOOD

CLITORIS

LABIA MINORA

the available sensations. This also means that whatever happens later will be less satisfying than it could have been.

∿ Orgasm Redefined ∿

So, as we've mentioned a few times now, we recommend experiencing any sensual activity—whether you're with a partner or masturbating—by focusing your total attention on what is happening in the present moment. That is, resist any urge to think about the future or the past or your everyday concerns.

Sensuality is about enjoying each caress with all of your ability and feelings. When you slip into your head and start comparing the current experience to a previous one or wondering what will happen next, your attention is in your mind and not on the sensation at hand. As soon as you find yourself doing this, guide your attention back to what is happening in your body. When thoughts come into your head during meditation, the advice is to place your attention on your breathing in order to stop the thoughts from taking over. When thoughts come into your head during a sensual experience, instead of placing your attention on your breathing, place it on the physical sensation you are experiencing. (In Exercises 5A and 5B we describe how to verbally acknowledge good feelings, a technique that can help you to stay in touch with those feelings.)

Why do we as teachers of sensuality place so much importance on staying with the sensation in the present moment? Because doing so is key to our "new and improved" definition of orgasm. We believe (and have taught many students) that an orgasm can begin at or even before the first genital stroke. An orgasm really begins in the mind. Just as a man can have a wet dream without being touched, anyone can experience sexual pleasure deliberately, without touching the genitals. An orgasm can begin when you place your attention on your genital area and allow yourself to feel all the wonderful sensations that occur there naturally—and to approve of the sensation even if it is only a little tingle or a slightly warm feeling.

Take a moment and focus all of your attention on the good feelings in your genitals. Uncross your legs. Just take a moment. There are a lot of nerve endings ready and waiting for you to notice them. The more you approve of the positive sensations that are happening, the better you will feel and the more easily you will notice them in the future. Once you are able to feel these good sensations just by deciding to do so, you will realize that orgasm is actually our natural state and that one has to be thinking about something else to distract oneself from the good feelings that are readily available. This natural orgasmic high isn't the same as what we call a "massive" orgasm, but once your genitals are stroked in the right way it can turn into one very quickly.

Much of the emphasis in our previous books was on teaching readers how to have a long, fantastic orgasm. Equally important—but perhaps less flashy than an extended orgasm—is the possibility of starting an orgasm on or even before the first stroke. Most people believe that a certain number of strokes or a certain length of time is required before an orgasm begins. This is commonly called the arousal period. In fact, we have found that people do not have to wait in order to start feeling pleasure. We have found that people who believe they can achieve orgasm right away and who have practiced our techniques with partners and with masturbation are able to feel actual orgasmic sensation

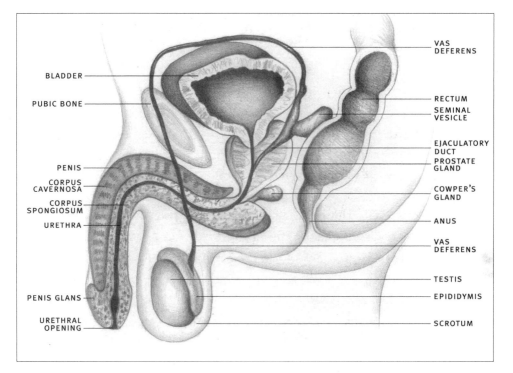

FIGURE 5.3. Male anatomy

on the very first stroke. What they are experiencing is not just arousal; it is the beginning of an orgasm. It is really amazing what human beings are capable of once they are aware of the possibilities.

The difference between the two types of orgasm lies in one's belief that it is possible to feel orgasmic on the first genital stroke, and also in one's ability to relax, focus, and feel. As long as a person is tensed up and waiting to get to the "point of no return" or waiting to feel better than they feel right now or

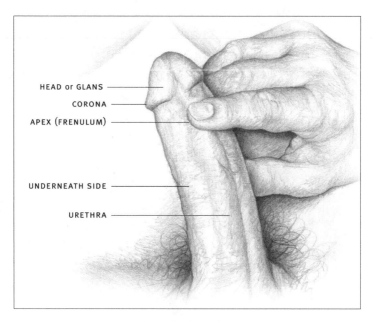

HEAD or GLANS
CORONA
APEX (FRENULUM)
UNDERNEATH SIDE
URETHRA

FIGURE 5.4. Underside of the penis showing the apex

waiting for what they previously thought of as an orgasm, they will be unable to feel all the exquisite sensations their body is experiencing at every instant.

When most people think of orgasm they usually think of male ejaculation. Most women have never seen other women have an orgasm, so they base their conception of orgasm on what they've heard all their lives denotes the end of the sex act: the man's ejaculation. A man's ejaculation is usually preceded by an arousal period during which he is not ejaculating. The problem with this paradigm is that ejaculation and orgasm are not equivalent. This is true not only for women but also for men. We define ejaculation as the *end* of the orgasm—not as the orgasm itself.

Most women do not ejaculate, and even when they do (a phenomenon known as female ejaculation), it is not necessarily as pleasurable as it is when a male ejaculates. That's because female ejaculation doesn't involve the clitoris and doesn't stimulate any pleasure or nerve receptors. Therefore, since women understand that they can be orgasmic without ejaculation, we have found it easier to train women in how to rethink their definition of orgasm. We have worked with hundreds of female students, all of whom had the ability to feel pleasure on the first stroke of the clitoris. At what point, then, is this pleasure classified as an orgasm? The answer to this question is really quite subjective. We say that as long as a person can appreciate the first stroke and any that follow, they are experiencing an orgasm. This does not mean that every stroke is the high point or climax of the experience. Hopefully the orgasm builds and goes higher and higher, with ups and downs along the way. At some point it will either stop or begin to go lower and lower, although involving ups and downs along the way down, too.

As long as a person remains in a relaxed state and is open to all pleasurable sensations, he or she will be experiencing an orgasm. Humans have long underestimated the ability to feel and experience pleasure. Accordingly, the orgasmic experience does not have to be limited to only a few moments of time and only a handful of contractions. All of the women whom we and our associates have trained are able to enjoy the orgasmic experience for many minutes, if not hours, and for hundreds, if not thousands, of contractions. They all can feel pleasure starting from the very first clitoral stroke. To call this state merely "arousal" is looking at the glass as half empty, a viewpoint that is unworthy of this magnificent capability.

Let's talk more about the importance of relaxation. Most people, both men and women, follow the male paradigm, in which one must tense up one's genitals while they're being stroked. This is necessary to reach a "point of no return," when the body goes into a convulsive mode that is defined as an orgasm. Vera likes to call these short, tensed-up orgasms "crotch sneezes." Once the ten seconds or so of intense pleasure is over, the person prefers not to be touched for a while. Most young men don't want to be touched at all for at least twenty minutes after ejaculating. As men get older, the refractory period gets longer and longer. Some women have a short, tensed-up orgasm and can then have another short orgasm after a brief refractory period; these are referred to as "multiple orgasms."

Our approach is different. The major difference is that instead of tensing the body, one must relax as much as possible without falling asleep. Then the orgasm begins with the first genital stroke or before, and continues for as long as one desires to be touched. With some practice, when one learns to relax and feel every stroke and also to acknowledge the pleasurable feelings, the sensations become more intense sooner. Once a person has reached the point of being able to fully relax and feel every stroke, he or she will experience sensations for an extended period of time that are at least as strong as those produced by tensing up the body in anticipation of those final ten seconds. What the person is experiencing is a real orgasm, with all the signs attributable to orgasm, including contractions, engorgement, lubrication, flushing of the face and neck, increased heart rate, sweating, and of course pleasurable sensations—only it lasts and lasts. This is what we define as an extended massive orgasm, or EMO.

Sometimes a person who is learning to have an EMO can feel frustrated if they focus their attention on the outcome rather than on the sensations. Some people wonder if they will ever again enjoy the intensity of sensation they used to experience when they tensed up during sex. We advise those students to be patient and to approve of as much sensation as they can during each moment of stimulation. Getting to the point where you feel these intense bodily feelings takes practice, and some folks have to practice more than others. Another idea is to practice being relaxed for a while and then revert to the old habit of tensing up before experiencing the powerful crotch sneeze at the end. We like to think of ourselves as offering something new to people without taking anything away. We are just adding some new tricks. If a person sticks with the relaxed method, eventually the sensation they experience will become more powerful for much longer. Some people adapt easily to the relaxed method; they take to it like ducks take to water. Others are more resistant and take to the new technique like cats take to water. They may have to practice for a longer time before they feel a significant increase in intensity of sensation.

A few more words about skillfulness in bed. If a person is truly confident about their abilities to pleasure and be pleasured by another person, they do not have to brag about being a great lover. Other people can sense true confidence. Keep in mind that if you are planning to make love with someone new for the first time, you do not want to put extra pressure on them to have a great orgasm just because you've been exposed to our teachings about how to do so. Nor do you want to imply that you know more about the other person's body than they do. The most important thing is to have fun, be playful, and enjoy the time in bed together. You can plan and talk about doing certain activities, but in general you should play it by ear and do only what feels good. It is usually better to do too little than to go too far, since you do not want to scare off your new lover and cause him or her to resist going to bed with you again.

∼ Fantasy ∼

It is tremendously important to be able to talk with your partner while receiving and giving pleasure. (See Exercise 5B for some training in how to do this.) In addition, talking about your fantasies and listening to your partner talk about his or hers can increase the fun and sensuality of any sexual experience. Almost every person whom we have met or who has studied with us has indulged in some kind of sexual fantasy at one time or another. Some people have less of a fantasy life than other people do, but everyone fantasizes at least occasionally.

When Vera is having an EMO, she reports that her attention is on what she is feeling rather than on any fantasy. Other women whom we've talked with fantasize almost constantly during the throes of a fantastic orgasm. As long as the person is using the fantasy to feel more and not simply to escape into head thoughts, we think it is okay to fantasize during lovemaking. At the same time, if the orgasm is intense and the pleasure is great, it is certainly okay to skip the fantasy.

Fantasies can vary from realistic scenarios to far-out imaginings that have no chance of ever happening. We have had students who've fantasized about being pleasured by four-handed and four-legged alien creatures or about having sex with wild animals, like panthers and tigers. We have known heterosexual students who've had homosexual fantasies. This is unusual for men because for a man to admit to fantasizing about other men is more taboo than for a woman to do so. Homosexual men, however, do fantasize about other men.

Men tend to have more realistic fantasies. They may think about a former lover or about a woman they saw earlier that day who was wearing a revealing outfit. Men's fantasies are often very simple, without much of a story line. They may be tantalized by thinking about a specific part of a woman's body, like her butt or leg or breast. The fantasy usually involves little if any talking; the woman is often doing things to him that he has done before or would like to have done to him. Some men may fantasize that they are having their way with a woman. We have known men who've had voyeuristic fantasies; that is, they see themselves watching another couple making love and perhaps doing some wild things. Both men and women fantasize about doing it with multiple partners simultaneously.

Women usually create more of a story to go with their fantasies. Their imaginings may include dialogue, a plot, and costuming. Women often fantasize about being another person's pleasure victim: having someone court them, romance them, and perhaps have their way with them sexually. Unlike most men's fantasies, naked body parts and the actual sex act may or may not be a part of a woman's fantasy. Sometimes women fantasize about an ex-lover, an acquaintance, or a famous actor like Paul Newman or Brad Pitt (depending on her age). Or they might fantasize about a dashing pirate figure or about being followed on a train by some unknown gentleman.

The ability to express oneself with one's partner while having sexual thoughts about things or people besides the partner allows a person to be more exposed and therefore more revealed and more real. Although expressing oneself this way can be scary, it also creates the possibility for more intense sensations and feelings. To be embarrassed and ashamed of one's thoughts and fantasies can metaphorically thicken one's skin to the point where the ability to feel is diminished.

At the same time, it is probably better for two people to wait to talk about their respective fantasies until they have been in a relationship for a while. As a good rule of thumb, you may not want to talk about another woman or man, including exes, when you're about to go to bed with someone new for the first time—or the first few times, for that matter. The newness of the experience will create plenty of excitement. The encounter itself will be like fantasy. If you are fantasizing about something that doesn't relate to your new lover, keep it to yourself at this point, but at the same time feel all right about having the fantasy. Sharing any fantasies you may have about your new partner—for example, talking about doing something naughty with him or her—is okay if doing so turns both of you on.

I like to fantasize when I am the person receiving the pleasure. My fantasy might be as simple as thinking about my partner's thighs, legs, butt, or feet touching my genitals. When I get to express that my fantasy while she is stroking my penis with her hands, it can add to my turn-on. The fantasy is about her, so she won't be jealous over another part of her body that I find sexy. My partner needn't change anything she's doing, but if she says something, like she is going to run her legs and calves over my penis, it can increase my fun and level of sensation.

Once you have been in a relationship with someone for an appreciable amount of time, it may be okay to learn what their fantasies are and to discuss yours with them. This doesn't mean you necessarily want to do the things each of you fantasizes about; the shared thought is itself a turn-on. If you know what type of fantasy turns your partner on, it can be fun during a sensual experience to play with them in a way that's related to that fantasy—again, not necessarily acting out the fantasy but merely talking about it. Likewise, when it is your turn to be pleasured, you can express some of your fantasies, which your partner can use to create more pleasure for you. Remember, men and women have different kinds of fantasies, so just because something turns you on, it may not do the same for your partner. By talking with your partner and paying attention to him or her you will learn what kinds of things they like to talk about and what they do not.

Sometimes it can be fun to enact a fantasy, but usually just talking about it will do the trick. I have engaged in a number of *ménages à trois* (threesomes) over the years. You may be surprised to learn that the actual pleasure I got from these encounters was less wonderful than the fantasy about them. It is almost every man's fantasy to go to bed with more than one woman at a time, yet for me the experience wasn't as good as being with just one woman. That's because one of the women was usually more fun than the other, yet I felt obligated to pay somewhat equal amounts of attention to each of them. This distracted from the pleasure I would have had with the more enjoyable woman had we been alone. Furthermore, there is potential jealousy over who gets more attention from me, who gets to touch the penis, and who gets to be the one to squirt me. Don't feel too sorry for me; it was still usually a fun experience, highly erotic, and available for fantasy material later on.

~

Now that you are in bed and have decided to go for it, hopefully the information provided in this chapter will prepare you for a wonderful time. You will become a better lover by knowing about the significance of being in the moment, relaxing, expressing your feelings, and using your integrity; the importance of female engorgement; the ability to get the most enjoyment out of each genital stroke; and how to use fantasy to your benefit. The remaining chapters provide even more techniques for being the best lover possible.

But first, the following exercises show you ways to learn exactly how to touch your partner—and also ways to get your partner to touch you exactly how you want to be touched.

✧ EXERCISE 5A ✧
Sensual Acknowledgments

This is an easy and fun way to practice your appreciation and acknowledgment skills. You can perform the exercise almost anywhere you eat, but you'll get the most out of it if you do it when you are enjoying a special meal, either at home or in a restaurant.

Instead of just gulping down your food, first take some time to delight in the food's aroma and appearance and to comment about what you smell and see. Next, deliberately linger over each bite, savoring all the wonderful flavors. Make comments of appreciation between swallowing and sinking your teeth into the next bite. Pretend that you are a food connoisseur or gourmet. If you have wine or another beverage, express your gratification as you sip it. Throughout the meal describe the flavors, textures, aromas, and presentation in as much detail and with as much pleasure and creativity as you can.

If food is not your thing, you can do this exercise in a garden. Take time to really look at and appreciate all the beautiful plants—their textures, colors, and fragrances. Describe what you see and smell in as much detail as you can.

✧ EXERCISE 5B ✧
Sensual Touch and Communication

Keep the lights on and your eyes open for this exercise. When you and your partner are in bed, select one of you to be the toucher and the other to be the touch recipient. The touch recipient then chooses a part of the body, other than the genitals, that he or she wants touched. It can be the inner thigh, the neck, the breast, the stomach—whatever.

Toucher, before touching the recipient, begin by announcing in advance what you are going to do—then do exactly and only that. The object is to make it as safe as possible for the touch recipient. Continue to announce everything in advance; that is, before changing the stroke or even before removing your hand, tell your partner your plans, and stick to them.

Meanwhile, touch recipient, verbally acknowledge what you like about the touches. Make your comments as specific as possible. Any positive statement will do; for example, "That feels good," "Love your fingers on my thigh," "You have great hands," or even "I could feel that stroke in my genitals." These are just examples; you will have to come up with lots of acknowledgments on your own. That is why we think it is a good idea to practice with food and other things first and *then* to perform this verbal appreciation on parts of the body other than the genitals.

Touch recipient, when you want to be touched differently—whether with more or less pressure, faster or slower, in a different area, with a different part of the hand, or with a different type of stroke—first give at least one verbal appreciation, then ask if your partner will "use more pressure," or "rub with your fingernails," or whatever. Ask for only one change at a time. As soon as the toucher moves in the requested direction, again verbally acknowledge your appreciation. Then start the cycle over with another affirmative statement. If the change is exactly what you want, let your partner know, and if it is not quite what you want, then restate your request nicely. Keep using this three-part sequence of a request sandwiched between at least two appreciative comments. You can always add extra acknowledgments anywhere in the cycle. Keep asking for what you want until your partner does it just the way you want him or her to do it.

Meanwhile, toucher, ask your partner questions that he or she can answer with a yes or with a no. Phrase the questions so that your feelings won't be hurt no matter how your partner answers. That is, avoid questions like "Does this feel good?" or "Do you like this stroke?" because although they can be answered with a yes or no, your partner may want to avoid hurting your feelings and therefore may decide to lie rather than to give a possibly hurtful response. Questions like "Would you like it harder?" or "Would you like more pressure?" are good ones. If the touch recipient answers no, ask a different question. For example, if they don't want it harder, maybe you can ask them if they would like it lighter, or ask about speed or location or type of stroke. When the recipient responds to a question with a yes, make the appropriate changes in small increments, and repeat the question until the answer is no. This way you will focus in on the exact stroke your partner wants. Also, remember to be careful not to change the stroke before asking permission or announcing the change.

It is more than okay—it is even necessary—to take deliberate breaks while in the process of touching your partner. Either person can call for a break. The toucher just tells the recipient that they are going to remove their hand and take a break. You may want to take a break to get into a more comfortable position, to talk about something that came up, because you happened to notice that your partner has stopped feeling, or just because you feel like it. The touch recipient can also call for a break for any reason. Just remember to verbally approve of your partner first. One note to the touch recipient: As long as the touches you are receiving continue to feel good to you, it is almost better to let your partner call the break, as you are learning not only to communicate but also to surrender.

This is a communication exercise. Later, when the communication is better and you know your partner's likes and dislikes, you will be able to change strokes before asking each time. Once you are more at ease and are used to talking while touching and being touched, you can move on to the genital area, where many of us have so much charge, and it will feel less challenging.

✧ EXERCISE 5C ✧
Adding the Genitals

Before starting this exercise, decide how long it will last. Have some lubricant handy. Get into a position where the person being touched is lying down and the person touching can see and easily touch the genitals. The position needs to be comfortable enough for the toucher to be able to stay in the same position for some time.

Begin as you did in the previous exercise, but use lubricant whenever touching the genitals. The person touching starts to stroke after first communicating what they will be doing. He or she asks yes or no questions whose answers will not offend either party. The person being touched verbally acknowledges the good feelings and asks to be touched as they desire. After the toucher moves in the direction of the request, the recipient rewards them with another verbal appreciation. Continue doing this for the agreed-upon length of time.

Toucher, at any point during the exercise you can add some verbal appreciations. Simply report on any signs of pleasure that you feel or see in your partner. It is very important when touching your lover's genitals to pay attention and make positive comments about what you notice in them. They will become engorged and change shape, size, and color. You will also notice sensations in your hands that are more pronounced than those produced by touching other parts of the body. It is beneficial to report these to your partner.

✧ EXERCISE 5D ✧
Sharing Fantasies

It can be fun to share your fantasies with your partner and to ask them to share theirs with you. Tell your partner what kinds of things turn you on. Let them know if you want them to role-play, or if you want them just to talk about certain things during sex. Revealing your respective fantasies can be quite exposing and can thus be beneficial to a couple, but it can also be quite scary, so only do this if you and your partner feel comfortable about it.

∾ *Chapter Highlights*

- ◆ To pretend to be in the throes of some sexually chemical intoxication if you don't actually feel it is counterproductive to the sensual journey.

- ◆ If a person is waiting for the "pleasure fairy" to come and rescue him or her, it may be a long wait.

- ◆ Zorba the Greek said it is a sin for a man to refuse a woman's offer to go to bed; however, once in bed he must do only what feels pleasurable and not do things simply because he thinks he should or because he feels obliged to.

- ◆ It is just as important to bring a woman's genitals to engorgement and readiness before intercourse as it is to engorge a man's penis.

- ◆ To most people, ejaculation is equivalent to orgasm and defines the end of the sexual experience. By contrast, we think of it as the *end* of the orgasm—not the orgasm itself.

- ◆ As a good rule of thumb, you may not want to talk about another woman or man, including exes, when you're about to go to bed with someone new for the first few times.

CHAPTER 6

Cherishing your open heart
To be my love,
To be the magic wand
That your desire inspires.
Take your bow and let me watch you,
As you gracefully attract
My ballistic attention
Toward your bending over.

Her Side of the Bed
News for Women on Achieving (and Giving) Pleasure

*T*his chapter explores how a woman can have a wonderful relationship with her man. Although the chapter is written as if we were speaking to women, men
can also benefit from much of the information included here. We describe the
powerful tool available to women of trusting their clitorises, how to civilize
men, how to understand why men lie, the proper training and reading of men,
and how to get the most out of a sexual experience.

∽ The Choice of Pleasure ∽

Compared to men, women have extra tools in their pleasure basket that can
help them in their intimate relationships. The best tool they have is the fact
that they are the source of life and of turn-on. As described in the first chapter,
turn-on is a woman's ability to influence men and other women with her
desires, both sexual and otherwise. Both women and men are necessary ingredients for reproducing our species, but only a woman can give life, and only
she can attract and turn a man on so that he responds with his attention and
his seed. It is the woman who signals that the time is right for pleasure and
lovemaking.

As we've touched on throughout this book, women have been second-
class citizens at least since the time of the agricultural revolution. Only in the
twentieth century have women begun to achieve partial social equality with
men. Therefore, women historically have had to resort to covert and under-
handed tactics to gain a measure of social equity with men. Although women
undoubtedly have suffered much from our patriarchal society's negative preju-
dice toward them, they also have been able to use their underdog status to gain
some leverage in the cultural battle of the sexes. As Susan Jane Gilman points
out in her book *Kiss My Tiara*, things have been getting better for women.
Five hundred years ago women were mostly serfs and peasants who held little political power (except for an occasional queen). One hundred years ago
women still could not vote, even though male ex-slaves could. Forty years ago
women could be harassed on the job and fired for getting pregnant. A generation ago, before the passage of Title IX, women hardly participated or received
scholarships in college athletics. In spite of being second-class citizens for so

long, women have not lost the battle of the sexes; if anything they have won most individual battles.

Almost every woman is angry at men for the reasons we described in Chapter 4. A relationship between a man and a woman will obviously fail to thrive if anger is the emotion *du jour,* day in and day out. A woman has to decide that a fun, pleasurable life is more important to her than her anger or revenge for the slights that men have inflicted upon women and upon her over the years. She has to decide to make friends with the enemy, teach him who she is, and be willing to expose her powers and her weaknesses.

How to teach a man who you are and how to train him to become a civilized human being are brilliantly described in *Mama Gena's Owner's and Operator's Guide to Men,* by Regena Thomashauer. The book details many examples of ways in which women have created wonderful lives for themselves and their partners. According to Mama Gena, knowing and asking for what you want, appreciating what you have created for yourself and your partner, and taking responsibility for your life are the main ingredients in the recipe for creating a winning relationship.

Women have a closer affiliation with pleasure than most men do. Men are more into success and production, while women, because of either biology or cultural factors or both, seem more inclined to make pleasure a higher priority. Still, because we live in such a pain-oriented society, as we described in our first book, *Extended Massive Orgasm,* even women aren't very pleasure prioritized. However, women will choose pleasure quicker than men will once they realize it is available to them free of cost at any time they choose.

The way to this boundless pleasure for a woman is via her built-in pleasure center: her clitoris. The clitoris is the only organ on the human body—male or female—whose sole function is pleasure. (A possible exception is the male nipple, whose pleasure potential is rather limited, compared to that of the clitoris.) We have noticed that when women fully come into their own as the powerful sexual beings they are, and when they get so in tune with their clitorises that they feel the full effect of the orgasmic potential that is available to them, they become free to savor life fully and to play the woman-man game with all their clout. And when a person goes in the most pleasurable direction each time a choice comes up, his or her life evolves to such a marvelous state that it will include success and everything else, in addition to pleasure.

∼ Trust Your Clitoris ∼

The best way we know of for a woman to decide whether or not a choice or an offer is pleasurable is to pay attention to her clitoris and trust it to guide her in which choice to make. When her clitoris feels good, a woman can feel confident going in that direction. When it feels less than good, she can either investigate the choice by asking questions and otherwise communicating, or she can decide not to take that path. When no apparent choice feels good, look for another one that does or realize that you are temporarily insane. We say "insane" because one definition of insanity is believing you have no reasonable choices, when in fact there are many possible solutions to every problem and every situation, and people are never limited to just one or two choices. Sometimes, however, we humans get stuck and cannot see all the choices. Although men do not have clitorises, they do have choices to make, and they too can get stuck with apparently no good direction to go in. If that happens, whether you're a woman or a man, it would be a good time to talk to a friend or a professional.

Here's an example of someone who ultimately made a choice that felt good to her, even though arriving at that decision was challenging at first. We have a friend who wanted to leave an abusive relationship. She thought she had to either stay married for the sake of her child or live close to her abusive ex-husband so their daughter would be near both parents. She felt as though she would lose with either choice. In fact, she did not have to stay in the same city as her ex-husband. She could move anywhere she wanted to. When, at the suggestion of a number of her friends, she finally moved across the country to L.A., she met a wonderful new guy. Furthermore, her daughter loved being bicoastal. She relished having two sets of parents and the best of two worlds.

There are always choices that feel better than others. There will be times, of course, when the choices feel less than pleasurable, such as when someone dies or is sick. You may feel obliged to go to a funeral or visit a sick friend even though you would rather do just about anything else. Because of our conditioning and who we are, sometimes we are better off following our obligations if doing otherwise would cause us to feel guilty or like a rotten person. In this case you can still follow and trust your pleasure center to guide you to make the perfect decision.

Some people believe that if they choose this hedonistic way of living, they either will end up destitute or will harm those around them. This is a totally erroneous theory. The choices guided by your clitoris will take into account the feelings of others. Poor choices are much more likely to be made when you decide with your head and avoid listening to your pleasure center. The more a woman feels orgasmically gratified and the more confident she is in her ability to receive pleasure, the better able she is to determine what she wants and to trust her choices. She automatically trusts her clitoris to guide her to the right decision.

Finally, it is useful to realize that you do not have to second-guess whether you made the right choice, because any choice you make is the right one. It doesn't matter all that much if you go left or right, as long as *you* believe you chose the right road. When the next fork in the road shows up, you can know that you will be able to make the right choice. You are not forced to go in any direction, and it is even okay to switch roads along the way if you feel that another one would be more fun or better for you in any way. Mistakes are only made in hindsight, and the more one is able to trust one's feelings of pleasure, the likelihood of making a wrong choice, even in hindsight, will be decreased.

Guilt arises from choosing to go down a certain road because of specific factors and then later (sometimes sooner than later) deciding it was a bad idea based on other factors. For example, maybe you were out with your friends having a good time and you saw an ice cream shop. You all went inside and you had a hot fudge sundae because it looked so wonderful, tasted so good, and was fun to indulge in with your friends. Then later maybe you felt guilty because you're feeling a little overweight and believe that ice cream has too many "empty" calories. You originally chose the sundae because it seemed fun and tasty, and later you felt guilty because you interpreted your choice based on your mind's placing more emphasis on other factors—in this case your worries about your weight. Guilt is a cheap thrill, but it is not a necessary part of living a wonderful life. It is there for the taking whenever you decide to have it, but remember that you are the one who creates it.

∾ Bear Training ∾

We jokingly call men uncivilized because without women around they would probably still be living in caves. Someone once said, "Men are like bears with furniture"—and some single men hardly have any furniture. Of course, not all men meet this description, especially some gay men, but enough of them do to allow us to generalize. Usually women are the ones who want to fill a home with comfortable and decorative furnishings and accessories—who want a nicely made bed, so to speak. When a woman moves into a man's home she adds cushions and curtains and other items to enhance beauty and comfort. Before women were allowed to serve in the armed forces, soldiers' barracks were very plain. They held only the bare necessities, such as a cot, table, and chair. Recently we saw some women soldiers and their living spaces on television. Their rooms contained pictures and other decorations, and generally looked more comfortable than the men's.

When Vera found me, I was living in a small space in a communal-living situation. My room was actually a crawl space that had been converted into a sleeping area. I couldn't stand up because the ceiling was too low. I slept on top of a soft rug with some sheets and a sleeping bag. I hung most of the few clothes I owned on some cross beams; the rest I kept on the floor. I didn't even have a chest of drawers. Luckily, I didn't sleep in this room too often, as I had a number of girlfriends. Vera, by contrast, had a nice bedroom with a closet and a chest of drawers and a bed and a nightstand. She slowly allowed me to move some of my stuff into her room.

As we have discussed, a woman wants everything. She wants a fun, scenic ride with lots of attention. On her own, a woman can have a great ride. However, taking someone with her can make it even more enjoyable. A beautiful sunset seems more exquisite when seen with someone else. And another person, if properly trained, can take you to a higher and more gratified place sexually than you can go by yourself. For a woman to get the partner she wants, as we pointed out in Chapter 1, chances are she's going to have to train him. But training and teaching one's partner are both the answer and the problem. They are the problem because sometimes it seems like too much work to invest all that time and effort into someone who you aren't even sure is the right one. Still, even if he turns out to be the wrong one, by getting him hip to who you really are and what your desires and goals are you will be doing yourself and him a big favor. You win because you get to play fully, with no hedging on your bets. He wins because he gains the information that women aren't inferior to him but are actually extremely powerful players and the only possible way to his true fulfillment. He gets to be a hero if it works, and if it doesn't, at least he will have learned some important lessons that he can take into his next relationship.

Of course, some men are a lot easier than others to become friends with and to open yourself up to, but it is for your own good as well as his that you are doing it. You may encounter some tough cases, where the guy's conditioning has made him so thick that just the thought of trying to train him is draining. If you don't want to get involved with a man like that, it's more than okay. If you feel this way, move on and find a better choice for yourself.

Sometimes it may seem that all the good ones are already taken. If you meet a man like that, as we pointed out earlier, it means some woman has already decided to put her love and energy into training him. Take heart: There are partially trained and practically untrained men out there who with a little love and a little polishing by you will look just as good to other women one day. Most men are full of untapped potential and will respond to a woman's desires if she treats him kindly and approves of his beingness. Most men, including married ones, feel so unapproved of by women that even a little bit of approval goes a long way.

We knew a lovely single woman who decided she was ready for an intimate relationship. She met a man at one of our communication groups who had never been in a serious relationship. He had an unkempt beard and wore shabby clothing—and we do not mean shabby chic. He had a job in the financial area but drove an old car and looked poor. To top it off he was obnoxious.

He acted as if he knew it all, and he was fairly sexist in his viewpoints. Anyhow, this woman saw some potential in him. She took him on, first as a research partner. They took sensuality-training classes together, and then she took him on as a romantic interest. She approved of him more than any woman had ever done before. They eventually got married. He got a better job and made more money. They had a beautiful daughter. They moved to a nice suburb outside of San Francisco and bought a lovely house. He dressed better, lost the beard, drove a nicer car, and became less obnoxious and less sexist. In short, he became one of those guys that other women saw as one of the good ones who were already taken.

～ Dogs Versus Bears ～

We affectionately titled the previous section "Bear Training." Most people are not used to training bears, but they are familiar with training dogs. Dogs respond best to approval and to rewards, such as biscuits. They do not respond well to beatings, yelling, or negative treatment. To train a dog properly one has to use lots of approval and to repeat every instruction over and over. Each time the animal behaves in a way that is in the direction of the goal, you immediately reward it. If you want your dog to learn to fetch, for example, you keep telling it, "Good boy," or "Good girl," or "Good dog" every time it succeeds. You carry around some dog biscuits and each time the dog picks up the stick and brings it back to you, you give it a goodie. You do not get mad at the dog or hit it for failing to bring back the stick. It will not learn that way. You keep repeating your instructions, show it the goodie, rub behind its ears—whatever it takes for your animal to succeed.

The same goes for training bears or for training people. Some men feel offended when we use the animal analogy or when we talk about a woman having to "train" a man. We say get over it—it is only an analogy. We aren't saying that men are dogs or as dumb as dogs or doglike. We *are* saying that using approval and positive reinforcement is simply the best way to train anyone, including women. As we've stated, most women aren't used to giving men much approval, but if a woman wishes to teach a man to be a better partner and friend and to treat her as she wants to be treated, then she will have to do what it takes. Even though many men are dumb (or maybe "unskilled" is a better word) when it comes to emotional and social interactions, they are still trainable. You may need to tell a man what you want more than once, and you have to understand that if you get angry at him when he fails, he will not learn as well as he would with lots of approval and rewards. When Vera married her first husband, her grandmother gifted her with a book on how to train a poodle, even though Vera had no dogs and did not plan to get one. Her grandmother was giving her what she knew to be the best information available on getting Vera's husband to treat her well and to be a wonderful partner.

Two movies that we recommend to our students contain great examples of women training men: *African Queen* and *Beauty and the Beast*, either the French version or the Disney cartoon. In both movies the woman gets the man (or the "beast") to change his beastly behavior by using patience, kindness, and communication. In *African Queen* Katharine Hepburn gets Humphrey Bogart to do her bidding by whatever means she can. Bogart plays a man who is negative, a drunk, and foul-mouthed. Hepburn plays a lady who is assisting her missionary brother in Africa. When the brother is killed, she must travel down a river to get away. The Bogart character has one of the only available boats, which she identifies as a way to achieve her goal of getting down the river. She sees his potential, so she overlooks his character flaws. She makes him the offer and he accepts, while grumbling about how impossible her idea is.

Hepburn has no doubt that Bogart will be able to do as she wishes. She knows she will have to occasionally "oil" him to get him into shape and to keep his motor running. She ignores his grumbling and doubts (see the section "Getting What You Want," below, for more about men's grumblings) and convinces him to go on this crazy adventure. They are confronted with one obstacle after another, including crocodiles, leeches, biting insects, Nazis, a broken motor, his fever, and a swamp area that has dried out, but because of Hepburn's clear focus on her goal and her expressions of gratification with everything Bogart does to overcome each obstacle, they become closer friends, more intimate, and a better team. At one point she pisses him off when she dumps his booze into the river, but after he sobers up, he forgives her and is actually grateful. When he is out of ideas, she helps him; for example, when he needs to fix the broken motor, she brings up the word "welding" in such a way that he thinks it is his idea. He gets to feel like a hero each time he triumphs over a mishap.

The two finally make it to the end of the river, where they are captured by a Nazi war boat and sentenced to die for being enemy spies. Before the scheduled hanging the captain asks if they have any final requests, and Bogart asks the captain to marry him to his beloved. The captain agrees and performs the marriage. Then the remnants of their little boat, the *African Queen,* to which they had earlier attached a makeshift torpedo, rams into the Nazi boat, exploding it, sinking it, and saving their lives.

In *Beauty and the Beast,* Belle, the beauty, is able to transform a monstrous creature into a well-groomed gentleman by using her love, sense of humor, loyalty, kindness, and lots of training. It is fun to watch these movies, and others that have a boy-meets-girl theme, with awareness about how the two genders relate to each other and knowledge about what it takes to have a successful relationship.

∼ Reading a Man ∼

People lie for two main reasons: either to avoid punishment or to impress someone. We all know of people telling whoppers to impress someone else. For example, a man may pretend to be richer than he is because he thinks women will be more receptive to him than if they think he is poor, or a woman will get a breast enlargement because she thinks big breasts will make an impact on a man. These sorts of lies often prevent people from getting to know the real you. Instead of creating a relationship they often thwart one from ever happening.

Lies told to impress people are quite common, but lies told to avoid punishment are even more common. They are also more dangerous to a relationship. Men usually lie to their partners to avoid being reprimanded if they've done something they feel guilty about and if they think their partners will be upset about it. When a person is proud about something, he or she doesn't withhold information about it. On the contrary, he or she is probably very vocal about it. A man thinks his woman will be upset about what he has done either because when he did a similar thing in the past she became furious with him, or because he's heard stories or seen movies or television shows about a man who did something comparable and as a result had to face the fury of a woman.

Because of men's nature, or for cultural reasons, most men are continually attracted to women—even men who are married, in a relationship, or single. In many Arabian countries the women are covered from head to foot to avoid sending sexual signals to men. Men are generally less selective than women about whom they would be willing to go to bed with. A good majority of men at least fantasize about this possibility even if they have no intention of acting on it. A man who denies his true feelings to his partner about other women because he fears her reproaches will hide this fact to the best of his ability. When a woman is able to understand that her man is just fantasizing because of his normal disposition, and when she feels good enough about who she is to allow him to express his erogenous feelings toward others, she will be way ahead in the game of having her man tell her the truth.

On the TV show *Ed* one of the married male characters was being pursued by a young college coed. He is having fun with her, and when she wants to kiss him and take him up to her room, he turns her down with some difficulty. Later he tells his wife that he went to the party with this girl, whom she had met previously, and that he was very attracted to her but nothing serious happened. His wife asks him what he means by that, and he tells her that the young woman invited him upstairs but he turned her down because he did not want to ruin a good thing with his wife. His wife jokingly says that he was a fool, that the girl is a babe and a half. He replies, "Yes, you're right, she is a babe and a half—but you're a babe and three quarters." His wife responds, "Good save." You can tell that what happened made the couple closer and more intimate and more in love than ever.

If the husband had been afraid to tell his wife about the incident and had withheld the story from her, the likelihood of its happening again with more serious consequences would have been higher than when he was totally open with her.

∼ Getting What You Want ∼

Your best tool for getting any man to do what you want is your turn-on and your "funability." A man responds quickly to real desire, especially if what you're suggesting sounds like fun and if he thinks he will win with you. You can make almost anything fun when you want to. Don't forget to reward good behavior and to let a guy know he is winning with you. Most of the time he doesn't have a clue whether he is winning or losing, but if he is getting any kind of sex, he believes he must be winning. He will probably continue to do what he is doing if he thinks his efforts are successful, so if you want more or better or whatever, you are going to have to tell him, maybe even more than once or twice. But tell him nicely so he can hear it.

When a man is presented with a request that seems difficult or that he has any kind of resistance to, he may groan or grunt or say no or get pissed or even start yelling. This is actually a good sign, for if he hadn't started thinking about how he is going to slay this dragon for you, he would probably stay silent. As Regena Thomashauer says, men are like big Mack trucks traveling down the road: It isn't easy for them to stop and change directions, and they make a lot of noise when they have to shift gears. His making noise means that he is already thinking of ways to give you what you want. Do not doubt your desire or his ability to fill it. Acknowledge your gratitude as if you already have what you want, and make him the cause for your gratitude. By this, we mean make clear to him that he is the one responsible for your wonderful feelings, and let him know how he is winning.

You are free to give him ideas if he requires them—either if he asks for help or if you covertly see something that will help. But refrain from pestering him with your request if you know he has heard you. The more you complain about how slow it is going, the slower it will be. It is your doubts that are slowing up the action. Know that you are wonderful, deserving, and totally attractive, and that you are the source of the energy he feeds on when he goes into action. Production only happens in the presence of appetite and desire.

The principles of how to get what you want are the same in bed as they are in other realms. A woman must trust herself to say yes to the specific sex acts she wants and no to those she does not want, no matter how much her partner may want to do them. If you do not want to swallow his semen or if you do not even want his semen in your mouth, these are prejudices you must honor. At the same time, it can also be beneficial to keep an open mind and to experiment occasionally with some new ideas and techniques. If something didn't feel good with a previous partner, it doesn't necessarily mean it will also feel bad with someone whom you may like more or who has more experience and better technique.

We want to devote a few more words to the topic of letting your partner come in your mouth. Some women like the taste of semen and others cannot stand it. Furthermore, the semen of different men varies depending on their diets, their cleanliness, and other factors they have less control over. You can ask your partner to experiment with different foods or to shower before going to bed to see if this will make a difference. Supposedly, adding sweet-tasting foods like pineapple to the diet and eliminating garlic and other strong, spicy ingredients will enhance the gustatory appeal of a man's semen. Still, some women just do not like the idea of someone coming in their mouth. In that case, one must be true to one's prejudices.

Most men want to pleasure women sexually, but if yours does not and you want him to, you could have a problem. You will either have to get him to learn how you like to be touched or find a new and better partner. Another option would be to do without fun sex altogether, but that is not the kind of relationship we're writing about. Because most men enjoy pleasing women sexually and in fact base much of their self-worth on their skills in bed, they should not be too difficult to teach. A man's ego might present a bit of a challenge, because it may tell him that he already is a great lover and has nothing to learn in the sexual arena. A woman can handle this situation by being fun and playful, by rewarding things she likes, and by asking in a friendly way for what she would like him to do. By discovering and rewarding a man for the things he does right and not finding him wrong for his past conditioning, a woman can get most men to treat her exactly the way she likes.

We think it is a good idea for a woman to know how desirable she is to men and also to be aware that most men want to give her pleasure and to fulfill her desires in and out of the bedroom. She will do well to ask for anything she wants, especially in bed, and to know that her partner wants to give it to her, whatever it is. Many women don't ask for what they want because they're afraid that their man will think they're too greedy or too wanton, but this is simply not the case. Almost all the men we have interviewed prefer for women to tell them what they want. As we wrote in Chapter 3, some women don't like to ask for what they want, hoping instead that their partner is a mind reader who automatically knows what they want. In addition, many women enjoy being overwhelmed, so the idea of asking a man for what they want causes them to fear missing out on this experience.

It might work to wait and see if your partner does what you want without your asking and if he overwhelms you in the process, but in the likelihood that he doesn't, it is best to tell him what you want and to ask for it in a friendly way. Once you have gone to bed with him a few times and have had fun (so that he feels successful with you), you will find that you don't have to direct him as often. You may also find yourself being pleasantly overwhelmed at times. You can now relax, lie back, and be more at effect (that is, receptive to pleasure).

∾ Follow Your Pleasure ∾

A woman first has to know what she likes and what feels good to her before she can tell a man what she wants from him in bed. We recommend to our women students that they explore their bodies by masturbating so they can learn what feels best to them (see Exercise 6A, "Self-Pleasure for Her"). They can experiment with lots of different touches, from light pressure to firm pressure and from fast speeds to slow speeds. Then they can take this new knowledge into the experience when they have sex with a partner. This allows a woman to give her partner lots of positive feedback about what she enjoys, and also to give him direct, easy-to-understand instructions. (See the exercises at the end of Chapter 5 for more about communication during sex.) It is also important for her and her partner to experiment and explore together. They can take turns touching each other and finding out the best ways to please and stimulate one another.

If you're interested in performing oral sex on your partner, know that there is no one right way to do it. Different men like different kinds of fellatio. You can experiment to see what you enjoy and what he likes best. You can lick his penis lightly with your tongue or put your whole mouth around it and suck with varying pressures. You can use your hands to stroke his penis, either while orally engaged or not. Ask your partner to report which touches and pressures feel best to him, and, again, only do what you enjoy.

Because this principle is so important, we want to remind you to touch your lover in a way that feels good to you, rather than to produce a certain effect in him. Touch your partner for your own pleasure and enjoy each stroke and each moment of contact with him, whether you are using your mouth or your hands or just cuddling. By doing it this way you will guarantee a fun time for both yourself and your partner. If she becomes a diligent student of pleasure, a woman can learn to feel her pussy and even to reach orgasm simply by placing her attention down there, without having to touch herself or to be touched (see Exercise 6B, "Connecting Your Clitoris"). Then when she's rubbing on a man or giving him a blow job she can take orgasmic pleasure in her own genitals at the same time. For your guy to know he is so much fun to touch that you are getting off while doing it to him will create that much more turn-on for him.

Do not be embarrassed to ask your partner to use some kind of lubricant when he rubs on your clitoris with his hands. You cannot rely on being sopping wet each time you have sex; furthermore, the clitoral area has fewer moisture-producing glands than the vaginal area. The techniques we teach, especially for extended massive orgasm, can involve stimulating the clitoris for long periods of time, in which case it is essential to use enough lubricant to prevent abrasion.

One more observation: We have noticed that a woman takes more enjoyment from playing with her partner's penis if her clitoris has been stroked and pleasured beforehand. This way she won't feel needy and can be more generous when she gives her man pleasure. On the other hand, sometimes a woman may want to just give her man some pleasure, focusing her full attention on him without first being touched. It is still a good idea to masturbate first so you will feel more generous and will be able to take more pleasure when touching him.

∾ To Bed? ∾

The question of whether or not to go to bed is ultimately up to the woman. She has to vote yes to complete the transaction, since most men will have already voted yes. Women often tell us they find it difficult to experience much pleasure during sex when they are not in love with the person. First of all, no one has to have sex with anyone he or she doesn't want to have sex with, and, second, it is nice if one at least likes the potential partner. Having said that, it is also true that a woman can experience intense pleasure with someone she isn't seriously involved with or in love with. A woman can experience wonderful pleasure with anyone if she is confident in her ability to feel and is able to surrender to her pleasure. It is a matter of deciding to go for the fun at hand instead of thinking that one is doing something wrong or believing the propaganda that one has to be in love to enjoy sensuality. It is also freeing to a woman to know that she can be pleasured without having to have intercourse or even any kind of penis contact.

All kinds of ideas and rules exist about how long a woman should wait before having sex with a new man in her life. We do not believe that people should live their lives according to anyone else's rules. It is safe to say that a woman's ability to communicate her desires and to be pleased in bed without having to have intercourse makes it less risky for her to go to bed early in a relationship. If you learn to experience sensual pleasure without believing that it must lead to intercourse, you are not going to get pregnant or get AIDS. Chances are, most men out there are quite ignorant about how to please you, although most will be willing and eager to learn as long as you give them lots of positive reinforcement. If you don't want to have intercourse, it is a good idea to explain this to a new man before going to bed, and to explain that you like it best when your partner manually or orally plays with your clitoris. If you like to play with penises, you can tell a prospective partner beforehand what you would like to do to him and to find out from him how he likes to be touched.

～ Genital Hygiene ～

Throughout our years of teaching we have discovered that many women (men too) have crotches that do not always smell like a rose, to put it politely. Most men won't tell you that your genital area smells, but they may subsequently refrain from getting close to it. If you are expecting to have a sensual interlude, it is probably a good idea to first shower and clean your genital area with soap and water, especially if you are unfamiliar with your partner's tastes.

In many parts of Europe they have bidets for cleaning the crotch area, but we in the United States have not advanced that far in our plumbing. It is so much more fun for a man to lick and touch a pussy that smells and tastes good than one that does not. On the other hand, many women do have wonderful-smelling genitals, and to hide their fragrance with too much soap or perfume would be a crime. Once a couple has been together for a while they can discuss sanely whether either partner would benefit from a shower.

～ Penis Size ～

Many men are hexed about penis size. They worry that they are undersized and therefore less potent in bed than a man who has a bigger penis. Most women, at least the ones who are orgasmically gratified, do not care about the size of their lover's penis. When a woman is relaxed and in an orgasmic state (or what others might call an aroused state—see Chapter 5 for our revised definition of orgasm), and when she has pushed out her vaginal walls, her vagina is collapsed around the penis. (See Exercise 6C for training in how to push out the vaginal walls.) When I give Vera a one-hour EMO in public, which we call a DEMO, the first half hour doesn't include any penetration. I then place my thumb about half an inch inside her vagina and ask her how deeply she feels it. She will report that she feels my thumb almost up to her navel, which in fact is about seven or eight inches away. This definitely proves to the audience that a man does not need a large organ to give a woman the most advanced pleasure possible.

A woman who is angry at a man may resort to using his insecurity about his penis to put him down and poke fun at him. But the reality is that the vagina is not equivalent to the penis; it is the clitoris that is homologous to the penis in terms of its potential for sexual stimulation. The vaginal wall houses few if any nerve endings, and no matter how big the penis is it probably still will not make contact with the clitoris during intercourse.

~

Women, we hope this chapter has demonstrated that by going for your own pleasure at all times, especially in your intimate relationship, you will cause your man to feel like a winner and to want to do your bidding. He can only win if you are happy, and the only way you can be really happy is to go for your pleasure.

The next chapter talks directly to men, hipping them to some basic things they should know about relating to and pleasuring a woman.

✧ EXERCISE 6A ✧
Self-Pleasure for Her

Many women masturbate, often to relieve physical pressure and tension. That is a good thing, but in this exercise we are going to build sexual energy or tumescence rather than try to get rid of it. The goal is for each stroke and each moment of the experience to be fun, pleasurable, and perhaps educational.

Make sure you are in a safe environment where you will not be disturbed by a lover, friend, or family member. Hang a "do not disturb" sign on your door if necessary, and make sure the telephone ringer is turned off. You want to dedicate this time to yourself and your pleasure. Start by making your space special, just as you did for the "visiting dignitary" exercise in the first chapter. Make sure you have something to drink, your favorite lubricant, and a towel or wash cloth to wipe yourself clean. It can also be beneficial to have a hand mirror available to further investigate how your genitals change and engorge with attention and touching.

Lie down in a comfortable position, and begin by touching yourself in different erogenous zones, such as your nipples, neck, thighs, the lips of your mouth—anywhere that feels good to touch. (For now, avoid touching your genitals; we'll get to them in a moment.) To increase your sexual energy use a light and quick touch. Try other kinds of touches, too; be creative. Using the mirror, see how your genitals look before you start touching them. Now start playing with your genitals, again touching lightly around the whole area in any way that feels good.

Place some lubricant on your hand and lubricate your inner vaginal lips, perineum (the area between your anus and vagina), and introitus (the opening to your vagina). Expose your clitoris with your other hand and put some lubrication there, too. Start stoking on your clitoris in a way that feels pleasurable. Use a repeated, reliable stroke. Remain as relaxed as you can. If you find yourself tensing up, take a break and relax again. As long as it feels wonderful, keep stroking your clitoris.

As soon as you sense that the next stroke will be less wonderful, either take a break or change the stroke. This will cause you to peak, which occurs when you have reached a high point, and deliberately come down so you can go up again. The break can be for a split second or for as long as you want. During your break you can take a drink or even look in the hand mirror to see what changes have occurred.

After your break, start stroking again, using either the same stroke you used before or a different one. Again, be creative. Experiment with all kinds of strokes, pressures, locations, and speeds. Each peak uses only one specific stroke. Just as in a mountain range there are lots of mountain peaks, you can produce as many peaks as you like. Just stay relaxed. You aren't trying to get anywhere, and by staying relaxed you will be able to feel more. You will also avoid going over the edge and having a "crotch sneeze."

When you're ready, you can bring yourself down (detumesce) by touching with slower and firmer pressure, both on your clitoris and on the surrounding area. You have built up a lot of sexual energy, so take your time coming down. Use the towel to wipe yourself off, which can bring you down further. When you are finished with the exercise, just tense up and release if you still want to have your old-fashioned orgasm. This kind of orgasm also detumesces you, as you will not want to be touched afterward.

✧ EXERCISE 6B ✧
Connecting Your Clitoris

A woman can connect the lips of her mouth as well as the inner lips of her vagina (labia minora) to her clitoris. She can actually connect much of her body to her clitoris, but it is easiest to do with erogenous zones that, like the clitoris, are made of erectile tissue. (Men, too, can learn to connect much of their body to their penis.)

Start by masturbating on your clitoris with your preferred lubricant until it is engorged and feeling real good. Then place a little lubricant on your other hand, and use it to start stroking on a second area, such as the lips of your mouth, while continuing to rub your clitoris. The strokes for the two different body parts should be very similar to each other in pressure, length of stroke, and speed.

After stroking both areas simultaneously for a while, remove your hand from your lips (or whatever body part you've been touching) for a few seconds, while continuing to stroke your clitoris. Then return your hand to your lips, and again rub both areas at the same time. Next, take your hand off your clitoris for a few seconds while you continue stroking your lips; then put your hand back on your clitoris and resume stroking both areas. Alternate removing and replacing each hand a number of times. When you do, notice if you experience any sensation in the area that is not being touched; if you do, wait to put your hand back on that spot until the sensation has diminished.

At first you may not feel much sensation in an area when you stop touching it, but even a faint stirring or a little heat is a positive sign. If you practice doing this exercise, you will feel more and more sensation each time until you can actually experience wonderful sensations in your pussy when you are kissing your partner or in your clitoris during intercourse due to the connection you've established between your clitoris and your labia minora.

〜

✧ EXERCISE 6C ✧
Pushing Out

A technique that is very beneficial to both women and men is called the "push out." Women have a figure-8-shaped sphincter muscle, the pubococcygeal muscle or PC muscle, encircling the vagina and the anus. On men, the same muscle encircles the anus and the base of the penis. This is the muscle that some sex experts and doctors teach their clients to strengthen with Kegel exercises, which involve alternately contracting and releasing the muscle. We do not teach our students to do Kegels, but we do teach them to push out.

To push out, simulate defecating and urinating at the same time, hopefully without actually doing so. For this reason, make sure that your bladder is empty before a sensual experience. Push out for only a second or two, and then consciously relax. Pushing out actually helps you relax, which enhances your EMO. The normal way most people experience orgasm is by tensing up the PC muscle, but in truth the way to feel the most sensation is to relax, which pushing out helps to accomplish. A further benefit of pushing out, when it is done properly, is to cause the vaginal wall to virtually collapse, so that instead of being balloon-like, the vaginal cavity is slightly longer and more cylindrical, and the opening to the vagina is less tight.

Because the vaginal cavity is both elongated and narrower when it is pushed out, there is less chance that the penis will bang against the cervix during intercourse. Furthermore, the fit for the penis will be much snugger on all sides, and it won't be strangled at the opening. As we discussed earlier in the chapter, this means penis size needn't have any bearing on the extent to which a woman feels "filled up" during intercourse. This technique is also good if a woman has intercourse with a man who has an extra-long penis, as a pushed-out vagina can accommodate a long penis without its hitting the cervix.

～

∽ *Chapter Highlights*

◆ The clitoris is the only organ in either human body—male or female—whose sole function is pleasure.

◆ The more a woman feels orgasmically gratified and the more confident she is in her ability to receive pleasure, the better able she is to determine what she wants and to trust her choices.

◆ We jokingly call men uncivilized because without women around they would probably still be living in caves.

◆ Another person, if properly trained, can take you to a higher and more gratified place sexually than you can go by yourself.

◆ And finally, to repeat a bit of wisdom from Chapter 3 (because it fits so nicely with the theme of this chapter), if you want to be loved you have to be lovable, if you want to be adored you have to be adorable, and if you want attention you have to be fun.

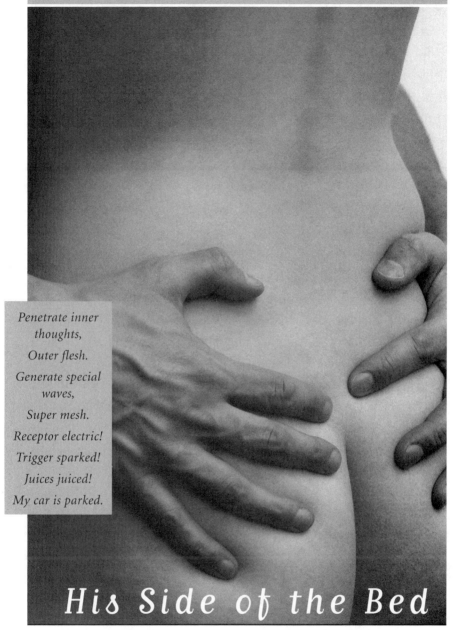

CHAPTER 7

Penetrate inner
thoughts,
Outer flesh.
Generate special
waves,
Super mesh.
Receptor electric!
Trigger sparked!
Juices juiced!
My car is parked.

His Side of the Bed
News for Men on Giving
(and Achieving) Pleasure

*T*his chapter is directed to men, although women can also benefit from reading it. It addresses the causes of penile engorgement; it offers detailed information about the clitoris and how to touch it, including touching someone who has never been touched there before; it discusses "castration," the rather harsh term often used to describe a man's feelings of impotence when he thinks he is losing with a woman; and it deals with the myth of women's insatiability.

∼ Penis Politics ∼

Penises would make lousy politicians because they don't lie. The simple fact is they engorge with blood when there is some female interest in them (assuming the penis's owner is heterosexual). Of course, a man can get his own penis hard by touching it or by fantasizing about something that titillates him. Otherwise, however, the only reason for a penis to rise to the occasion is when a woman is thinking about it or is having sensual thoughts and is sending the man signals—either through pheromones, gestures and body language, or some other kind of communication—whether she's conscious of doing so or not. Exactly how a woman communicates her sensual interest or desire to a man is still unknown. Any woman or girl who likes herself enough seems to be able to do it. She doesn't have to be a witch or to have any special powers.

If you ask a man to raise his right hand he will have no difficulty doing so. But if you ask a man to make his penis erect, he will have great difficulty performing this request on demand. We have been in a number of classes, as either teachers or students, in which a woman was asked to make a specific man's penis erect, and she was able to do so, reportedly a lot more easily than he could do on his own. Furthermore, a man can be at a party, in a business meeting, or in a classroom and become engorged without wanting to. He may actually prefer that the thing go down yet be unable to will it down. The penis is not something that a man can voluntarily control.

So the good news is that for the most part men don't get their own penises hard. A normal, healthy man no longer has to feel inadequate if his penis is unable to rise to the occasion and perform whenever he thinks it should. A man only responds to a woman's genuine desires; he cannot force himself on her. (We're talking here, of course, about men with normal psychologies. Rapists, who are wired pathologically, get erections based on abnormal stimuli, such as the desire to hurt and control women.) Yet when many men hear this they think it is bad news. They believe that some kind of power has been snatched from them. They feel less in control because they are starting to realize the extent of power women can have over them. To me and to other men, however, this was wonderful news. It made sense that we actually had little control over that appendage, and now we knew why. Nothing had really changed; we had only gained knowledge that helped to explain what we had already observed was going on. The news is freeing because instead of feeling impotent and insecure a man can know the true nature of his little beast. He can then move forward and communicate productively with his partner.

Some liberated women realize this power of theirs and will readily admit to it, while other women are in denial about it or at least don't want to own it. We have heard many stories about women blaming men for being unable to get it up, leaving the man feeling like an impotent eunuch, when in reality his lack of an erection had nothing to do with his functioning but rather was all about the woman and her true desires. We aren't trying to make women feel bad or guilty by saying they are somehow to blame for a man's inability to get hard. We _are_ saying that the penis is a good barometer of a woman's true desires in bed. As we pointed out in Chapter 5, a woman may say she wants to have intercourse, but unless her partner has an erection there is little that can be done about it. In this case it is a good idea for the man to talk more with his partner and to ask her questions about what she is feeling and thinking and about what she really wants. A woman may say she wants intercourse when what she really wants is more loving attention paid to her body, especially her clitoris. This is when it is helpful for a man to summon his self-confidence, to exercise his integrity and consciousness, and to tune in to his lover. When the penis of a man who feels good about himself seems to be refusing to cooperate, he can tell his partner in a nice way that at this time it feels like it would be more appropriate to play with her genitals—or whatever is true. He would do well to avoid getting angry or defensive, or blaming her directly for his failure to perform. Again, anger is the enemy of turn-on, and often the reason why a woman loses interest in the penis is because of something that has pissed her off, possibly something her partner did or did not do or say. Maybe he made some dumb, sexist remark that turned her off. In any case, it is a good idea for him to find out what he said or did so he can either apologize or avoid going down the same road next time. If he pays her some loving attention, he may cause her to feel better and possibly to have some more use for his penis.

Sometimes when a man is in bed with a woman, the penis will become engorged and the couple will begin to engage in coitus, only to have the penis shrivel as the man loses his erection. The same thing can happen while the woman is playing with the penis with her mouth or her hands, not just during intercourse. The penis can go flaccid at any time. This happens either because the woman has changed her mind and decided (on some level) that she really isn't up for an up penis, or because her desire to have intercourse has become tainted by her doubts about her attractiveness, or by her anger over something her partner said, or even by a memory from her past. Bottom line: The woman's attention has gone elsewhere. The man's attention can go elsewhere too, but when this happens, it is usually because the woman's attention went away first, or because the amount of turn-on she was sending dissipated. In any case, it was her decision to stop the process, even though she may or may not be consciously aware of how it all happened and of her responsibility for causing the situation.

Kathy, a woman we know, was in bed with her boyfriend. They were having fun touching each other's bodies sensually. The boyfriend was turned on and hard. He got on top of Kathy, and as he started to penetrate her vagina with his penis, it lost its erection and became flaccid. He didn't know why it happened, so he thought something was wrong with him. What actually happened was that Kathy was happy playing and touching but was not ready for intercourse. She wanted her lover to keep touching her genitals but found it difficult to express herself and communicate to him in bed. Later, when they took one of our classes and we explained these phenomena, they understood what had happened. They have since gotten married and have learned how to talk to each other in bed and ask for what they want. He no longer feels impotent or inadequate.

Of course, certain physiological problems, such as diabetes or vascular disease, can cause a man to have difficulty reaching engorgement. But if a man is normal and healthy, the only reason he will become engorged is because a woman has some interest in him, and the only reason he will lose engorgement is because she has lost that interest. The lack or loss of engorgement is really no one's fault. It is the result of a lack of communication between the man and the woman. Although we believe that the woman is ultimately responsible for the penis's becoming either erect or flaccid, it is both parties' responsibility to understand how they may have influenced this occurrence. As Dr. Vic Baranco wrote, "An erect penis is bisexually owned."

∽ Express Your Pleasure ∽

So, as we've stated, the underlying cause for a loss of erection is a lack of (or at least a lag in) communication between the partners. Specifically, one or both parties aren't expressing or admitting the pleasure they are experiencing. Underacknowledged positive sensations often turn into doubt, then turn into anger, and finally result in unconscious and inattentive behavior because the person fails to understand why he or she is angry.

It is human nature to continue doing something when it seems to be creating good results. If you are rubbing someone's shoulders, you will keep doing so for a longer time if the person tells you how good it feels and that you are doing a great job. If they say nothing, you will probably stop earlier because you aren't sure if you're doing any good. It can be wonderful if your partner is a great communicator in bed and reports all the wonderful feelings and sensations she experiences, but do not wait for or rely on her to start talking. Women have grown up in the same society as you, and neither sex was taught to talk in bed. In fact, we all have been conditioned to avoid talking during sex, to do it in the dark, not to look, to do it under the covers, and not to talk about it afterward. This is insane if a person wants to experience real pleasure. Becoming a good communicator in bed is simple once a person can get past their conditioning and realize the benefits they will reap.

The most important kind of communication you can engage in while in bed is to report all the wonderful feelings and sensations you're experiencing and also the ones you notice in your partner. The likelihood of your penis deflating due to lack of attention and appreciation will decrease the more you and your partner verbally appreciate each other. The more freely you are able to talk about your feelings during a sensual activity, the more freely your partner will also be able to talk. Once you are both communicating easily and effectively, your level of pleasure will rise accordingly. When both parties fully express their pleasure and their feelings, you will know what great sex feels like.

~ Penisometer ~

As we've said, the penis is a remarkable indicator of whether things between a man and a woman are going well or otherwise. But remember, just because a man's penis is on the way up does not mean that the woman wants to have intercourse. Rather, it is an indication that she is enjoying receiving the man's attentions and interacting with him. Some women like to get a guy hard just to test their powers, and others do so because they might want to go to bed later—or at least to entertain the thought or fantasy. Sometimes it is appropriate to give a woman feedback that she is turning you on, especially if you know her well or are in a relationship with her, and other times, for example in most professional situations, such things are best left unsaid. It is fun for a man to be turned on and engorged even if the woman he's responding to has no real intention of doing anything about it. It only gets difficult for the man when he hasn't had sex in a while or is extremely horny for other reasons. It is considered rape to use your penis on an unwilling recipient even if the woman is the one who started you up.

Some women are afraid to turn it up around most men for fear of the man's acting in a way that the woman won't appreciate. She may be frightened that he will want to stick it in her when all she was doing was thinking about it. Some women may have been molested or raped when they were younger and so now keep a lid on their turn-on for fear of the same thing happening again. If this seems to be the case with a woman you're interested in, it would be a good idea to talk to her about her experiences and to let her know that you are there for her and will never violate her.

Women give obvious signals when they want to be touched, but if you are unsure, it is worth your while to ask. Once you get to be a skilled operator of her clitoris, it is more likely that she will want to have sexual interactions with you. When you are rubbing on a woman with your hands or using your mouth there is no actual need for an erection. Sometimes a woman will turn it up while you are touching her with your hands. It is usually a gentlemanly thing to let her know in a friendly way that this has happened. Sometimes I will teasingly say something like, "I can feel that you are having some nasty thoughts right now." Often you won't have an erection while rubbing on your partner. This is normal and okay. You can still tell with your hands and by how you feel in general whether she is appreciating your strokes or if it is time for a break.

∽ Become a Clitoral Expert ∽

Men, we cannot overstate how important it is to learn your craft as a giver of pleasure. You have to be able to read a woman's signals about how fast to proceed, how much to tease, and when and if to approach her genitals and her clitoris. A woman usually likes it when a man takes the time to touch and kiss her before diving for her genitals. She enjoys his attentions and his compliments. The more you can tease her and increase her feelings of desire, the more pleasure you will create for her and for yourself.

You can tease a woman with words or by using light touches in the appropriate erotic places and then withdrawing to a less erotic area of her body. You will do well to become a master of her tumescence—that is, to learn how to take her up and take her down at will. Generally, fast, light touches will take a person higher or tumesce them, while firmer, slower strokes will bring them down or detumesce them, but with the right intention any stroke can be used to go in either direction. Both going up and going down can be very pleasurable, and both are parts of an EMO. It is important to know at all times in which direction your partner is headed. Sometimes, due to her desires or to a lack of time, a woman may require a faster than usual approach to her genitals. Once you are skilled at making love, you will be able to determine how quickly to proceed, whether to take her up or bring her down, and when to change directions or stay the course.

Until you learn all the intricacies of touching a clitoris with your hands and really seeing what you are doing, you will be missing out on much of the pleasure available to her and to you. The clitoris is not as easy to make friends with as your penis. Your penis will welcome, without resistance, almost anyone who gets it hard. By contrast, the clitoris is a slippery little organ. It will dive into the body, hide under the hood, and avoid intimacy until you prove your skills at wooing it into surrender. It can be had, but if you expect to get to this point without looking at it, using proper lighting, you will have a long and difficult path. We had one student who wore a miner's hat in bed, with the light aimed at his partner's genitals. We do not go that far in our recommendations, but adequate lighting is essential at first. Once you become friends with a clitoris it will come to you almost as quickly as your penis would surrender to a turned-on woman. Once you know your way around a woman's clitoris, you will be able to play with it without looking at it. You will be able to kiss your lover or enjoy face-to-face contact with her while stimulating her genitals. That said, however, for the most intense EMOs, visual contact with the clitoris is still the best way.

Under the Hood

The hood of the clitoris can be a tight or loose covering, or anything in between. Some are thick-walled and some are very fine in structure. Some women have hoods that don't pull back, and others have scarcely a hood at all. Each woman is built differently, so the amount of pressure necessary to pull the hood back and away from the clitoris will differ from woman to woman. (See Chapter 5 for illustrations of a woman's genitalia.)

When manually stimulating a woman's genitals, we recommend always using lubricant, unless her pussy is so wet that lubrication would be redundant. Any of a number of techniques can be used to expose the clitoris from under the hood. You can pull back the hood with the thumb of the same hand that you will use to stroke the clitoris. If you're right-handed, place the thumb of your right hand along the left side (from the woman's perspective) of the clitoral hood, and move your thumb upward, thereby exposing the clitoris. (If you're left-handed, place your left thumb along the right side of the clitoral hood and pull upward.) If you've used adequate pressure, the hood should move with your thumb, leaving the clitoris revealed (see Figure 5.2 on page 125). The thumb is now firmly pressed against the clitoral shaft and the hood is less visible. This position makes for an excellent anchor, enabling you to get to the clitoral head with your index or middle finger. We call it an anchor because keeping your thumb pressed against the shaft prevents the clitoris from moving around and playing hide-and-seek.

After becoming fully engorged, the clitoris will usually remain exposed and the hood retracted until the engorgement dissipates. The thumb can remain against the clitoral shaft as an anchor and a guide for your fingers, or you have the option of removing your thumb once the clitoris is fully engorged and exposed. Either way, this can be a fairly difficult maneuver and may take some practice to get just right.

An easier way for a beginner to expose the clitoris is to use your free hand. Place either your palm or fingers on the pubic mound (above the clitoris), and push upward to expose the clitoris. You can use quite a bit of pressure here; just make sure it feels good to your partner. The problem with using your free hand to expose the clitoris is that doing so prevents you from using it to anchor the clitoris or to stimulate the introitus and inside the vagina. It also prevents you from employing your free thumb as a monitor to determine the strength of her contractions. Usually I place the thumb of my free hand at the base of the introitus and fan the fingers of that hand beneath her buttock cheeks (see Figure 7.1 on the next page). You can even ask your partner to use her own hands to pull back on her pubic area to expose her little jewel.

Whether you use the one-handed or two-handed method for exposing the clitoris, we recommend using the thumb of your "doing" hand as an anchor, as described above. This way, the clitoris is trapped—almost pinched, really—between the finger and the thumb so it cannot escape. Once the head of the clitoris visibly engorges and surfaces so that it is totally exposed from under the hood, you can relax the anchor if you wish. We also recommend that you hook your "doing" finger under the hood. Bend the finger at both the first and second knuckle so that it makes maximum surface contact with the portion of the clitoris deep under the hood as you maintain contact at all times between the tip of your finger and the clitoris.

Until you are skilled at exposing the clitoris and keeping it exposed throughout the orgasm, we recommend that you remain in a position where you can see what you are doing, so you can be confident that you are stroking

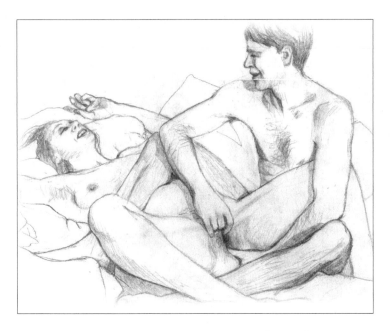

FIGURE 7.1. Doing a woman in the "primo" or
sitting position for a right-handed doer

directly on the clitoris. Again, staying in both visual and tactile contact with
your partner's genitals is the recommended way to produce the best possible
orgasm.

Upper Left Quadrant

The entire head of the clitoris, with over eight thousand nerve endings, is very
sensitive. However, the vast majority of women (about 90 percent) whom we
have trained or have talked to, once they are familiar with having their clitorises stroked, say that the most sensitive area on their clitoral head is what we
call the upper left quadrant. Imagine that the clitoral head is divided into four
areas, the upper left and right and the lower left and right. (The left side we
refer to here is from the woman's perspective, in the same way that her left arm
is on her left side.) Some clitorises are so small that it is almost impossible to
divide them into four areas, in which case your finger would be too big to stay
in one quadrant anyway. But on most women the clitoris is large enough to
envision four quadrants. In addition, with stimulation it will engorge to over
twice the size it is in its flaccid state.

This is valuable knowledge to have because a man who is able to keep stroking the clitoris in one specific quadrant, preferably the upper left, shows his partner that he is familiar with clitoral stimulation. (We have met the occasional woman who claimed that her upper right quadrant was more sensitive than her upper left. With a bit of experimentation you can find out what is true for your partner.) Once you have demonstrated your ability to stay in one quadrant and your lover is feeling intense pleasure and her clitoris is engorged with blood, the entire clitoris becomes even more available and you can move from quadrant to quadrant using whatever strokes you like. As long as you know which quadrant you are in and she knows that you know, you will have gained points in controlling her pleasure. Once the clitoris says, "Okay, you've got me," it will stay available for you to do with it whatever feels good to your finger.

How to Stroke

You do not have to continually stroke the clitoris throughout the orgasm, but you must be aware when you are on it and when you are not. For this reason it is highly beneficial to communicate with your partner at all times during the sensual act. She will be more able to surrender her nervous system to pleasure if you let her know what you are up to and what is going on. There is a big difference between deliberately removing your stroke from the clitoris while communicating that you are doing so, and having your partner wonder if you know that you're no longer touching it. A person cannot surrender her nervous system easily to someone she thinks isn't in control or who appears not to know what he is doing.

Once the clitoris is exposed, very short, up-and-down strokes are the best way to stimulate it to intense orgasm. This is because when the stroke is short you can stay on the clitoris for the whole stroke. When the stroke is too long you will be on the clitoris for only part of the stroke; for the rest of the stroke you will be either above or below it. Furthermore, a short stroke will allow you to stay in the upper left quadrant. This illustrates why it is so important to become visually acquainted with your partner's clitoris when you are first learning about each other's bodies—so you can see when you are on and when you are off target. This is also why it is vitally important to get your finger under the clitoral hood. A man who has mastery of a clitoris can touch any part of it at will and know exactly where he is.

Move the finger that is doing the stroking in an up-and-down motion as rhythmically as possible so your lover can surrender to your touch without feeling surprised by a constant switching of strokes. This is especially important while you are first touching her and getting her going. Once the clitoris is more engorged and she is having steady contractions, you can be less predictable with the length, direction, firmness, and frequency of your strokes. The best time to surprise her or to change the stroke is when you intend to peak her and then bring her down a bit. Sexual excitement tends to increase with a reliable stroke; when you change it or surprise the person, they tend to lose some sensation. Then, when you start a new, consistent, dependable stroke, sexual excitement can again increase. At the same time, however, stroking too much and for too long can also cause sensation to fade somewhat. That is why it is important to stay in communication with your partner. As long as her sexual energy is going up, any change will bring her down. If she is already going down, then the change will probably increase her sensation again. Whatever happens is okay, but if you have lost control of your partner's orgasm it would be best to do some talking.

This is the art of peaking someone and giving them an extended orgasm. It means you have to pay attention to your partner so you notice when she is going up, when she is about to go down, and when she is on her way down. Then, as long as you stay one step ahead of her, deliberately bringing her down before she is quite ready to go and taking her back up whenever you decide to, you will be able to control the orgasm and to take it higher.

The G-Spot

The term *G-spot* was coined in 1950 by Dr. Ernest Gräfenberg to refer to the spongy area at the front of the vaginal wall. Although there are no nerves at the surface of the vaginal wall, the front part of the vagina is near the area where the nerves from the clitoris enter the body. To stimulate this area, position one or two fingers on either side of the top of the vagina, as shown in Figure 7.2. Position the fingers with palm up, inserting past the first or second knuckle to a depth of one to two inches. Locate the spongy, bulbous tissue at the roof or

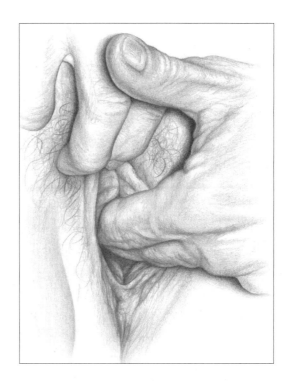

FIGURE 7.2. Two fingers of left hand inserted, just left and right of twelve o'clock

front of the vagina. This is the G-spot. Stroke the area by moving your fingers in a come-hither motion, feeling both the in and out strokes. We have found that some women like to be stroked at the exact center of the G-spot. Others find it uncomfortable to be touched there because the urethral canal runs through the area. If your partner doesn't enjoy being stroked in the precise center of the G-spot, stroke just to the sides of the center.

∾ EMO for Men ∾

Men can experience EMOs, too, and the principles for peaking a man and controlling his orgasm are the same as they are for women. As we described in Chapter 5, an ejaculation is merely the end of the orgasm, not the entire orgasm. A man's orgasm can begin on or before the first stroke, just as a woman's can. The more a man can relax and focus his attention on the pleasure he is receiving, the quicker and better will be his orgasm. If he is thinking about the ejaculation he hopes to have at the end of the experience, he will miss much of the orgasm that he could be feeling in the moment. We recommend reading *The Illustrated Guide to Extended Massive Orgasm* for a detailed description of male orgasm.

∽ How to Touch a Virgin ∽

If a woman is new to having her clitoris stroked, she may insist that it is too sensitive to be touched directly. (However, even many first-timers appreciate direct contact.) If she feels too sensitive, use a lot of lubricant and touch her very lightly, for only one or two strokes. Then take a break. Ask if she would like an even lighter stroke. It is better to err on the side of stroking her too lightly than too firmly. If you touch too lightly, she can always ask for more pressure, but if you touch too firmly, she will get defensive and will put her energies into not feeling instead of remaining open to as much sensation as she can.

Some women who claim their clitorises are ultrasensitive won't even touch themselves there; instead, they masturbate by rubbing on the clitoral hood. A woman can feel a lot of sensation by rubbing on the hood; however, to obtain a really intense orgasm it helps to touch the clitoris directly. If your partner remains resistant to being touched directly on her clitoris, one idea is to place extra lubricant on your finger and to let the lubricant act as a buffer between your finger and her clitoris. Your finger doesn't come into direct contact with the clitoris; only the lubricant does. For this reason we recommend petroleum jelly as a lubricant, because a dab of the stuff makes a fine "extension" to your finger when you're first touching a woman with an overly sensitive clitoris. This slow and safe approach will allow her to expand her willingness to be touched there, and by proceeding gradually and in small increments, eventually she will be able to accept more pressure and to be touched for more than just a couple of strokes. See the next chapter for more about this issue.

A woman with a sensitive clitoris may at first prefer a longer stroke. That's because during a longer stroke the clitoris is only being touched part of the time; for the rest of the stroke you're touching a less sensitive area, like her inner lips. By keeping the thumb of your nonstroking hand at the base of her introitus and applying fairly firm pressure there, you will be able to feel any

contractions, even small ones. If you can feel contractions and if it feels pleasurable and fun to keep touching her clitoris, this is your cue to keep stroking,
using short strokes if possible. As soon as you notice that the contractions have
stopped or faded, it is time to take a break. Let her know what you are doing,
and then start again. Touching her this way will cause her to realize that you
are in control and are using her pleasure as your guideline, which will make
her want to surrender to you that much more. Gradually she will be able to
extend the peaks of pleasure from three strokes to five, then to ten strokes,
twenty strokes, and then to a couple of minutes.

Remember that most women like a lighter pressure than most men do, so
find out how much pressure she prefers. This goes for other parts of her body
too, such as her nipples and breasts, which men often squeeze or bite much
harder than many women like. Again, no matter what part of the body you're
touching, it is always best to err on the light side and then to ask if she would
like more pressure. Clitorises, which are made of erectile tissue, are quite
strong and resilient. Once a woman is willing to surrender to her pleasure, it is
possible to squeeze her clitoris between your fingers with all or most of your
strength (depending on how strong you are), without causing any damage and
in a way that actually feels very pleasurable to her. This is not something we do
on a regular basis, but it is nice to know that the clitoris can take all kinds of
pleasurable pressures.

∾ Cunnilingus ∾

The art of orally stimulating a woman's genitals can be extremely pleasurable
and erotic. It is important that the woman whom you are pleasuring is a good
communicator so you will know that she is appreciating what you are doing,
and so you will know what she likes and what her preferences are. As is the case
when you're using your hands, it is important to use your mouth in a way that
feels pleasurable to you.

There are many different kinds of strokes you can use to stimulate a
woman's genitals with your mouth. You can vary the pressure and the speed.
You can use the tip of your tongue, the flat of your tongue, your lips, or even
place the whole clitoral area in your mouth and suck. Ask her before you start

how much pressure she prefers and her favorite speed and type of stroke. If she doesn't know, ask her to give you feedback while you are doing it to let you know what feels best. Make sure both of you are in a comfortable position. Use as many pillows as necessary to get the angles and the comfort level just right.

It is a good idea to start with a light touch, probably using the tip of your tongue. Now that you know where her clitoris is and how to pull back the hood to expose it, you can get your tongue right up under the hood and lick. If you know where her favorite spots on her clitoris are, you can tease her by first licking her lips, perineum, and introitus—until she is begging you to get to her clitoris. Use your hands to push up on the hood to expose the clitoris. Take time to look at it and to notice when it engorges. Take breaks and lift your head to visually take in the whole picture. Report how much fun you are having, and acknowledge the wonderful tastes and smells you are enjoying. Taking breaks also offers a chance to tease your partner even more. After a while her clitoris should become engorged and you will not have to keep moving her hood out of the way with your hands.

Because of your experience in getting her off manually, you will know when to peak her—that is, when to take a break or change your stroke. Some guys think they have to stay down there for a long time without any breaks in order to prove their endurance. This is not what fun and sensuality are about. Every stroke must be wonderful and precious, and to do anything because you are trying to prove something or to get somewhere in the future will lessen the experience.

As we have stated elsewhere, sometimes a person can have a bad taste or odor emanating from his or her genitals. If you are unable to enjoy putting your face down there, then it is vitally important to discuss this with your partner in a way that prevents her from feeling too hurt by the way you talk about it. (The same is true for women whose male partners practice less than pristine "crotch hygiene.") We have gotten a number of e-mails from women who were deeply hurt because their boyfriends found it too "smelly" to go down on them, and they did not know how to approach the subject with delicacy. Tell her how you really would love to give her oral gratification, and you think it would be a good idea for her to clean up first as you are very sensitive to smells—or something to that effect. Offer to get into the shower with her and make the shower a sensual experience. Unless a woman has a yeast infection or another STD, a simple, thorough bathing of the area will remove all offending odors.

∼ Blind-Spot Castration ∼

Women sometimes get revenge on their partners or hurt them by deliberately being unhappy in their presence. Of course, a woman may be generally unhappy and it will have little to do with hurting the man on purpose, although it still will have that effect. Many women are well aware, most of the time, of the unwritten contract that says the man is supposed to make them happy, and by being unhappy a woman causes her man to fail at this task. She may act miserable and by so doing actually become depressed. This causes the man to lose, which was her goal. She may be winning at one level, because she has achieved her goal of causing the man to feel like a loser, but she has done so at the cost of also causing herself to lose at something more important. It is like the old proverb that talks about cutting off your nose to spite your face. The only way a woman can really win in a relationship is by being happy, and if she's happy then the man will feel like a winner, too. Either both people win or both people lose; one cannot win while one's partner is losing.

When a woman is miserable and tells her partner that she thinks he is wonderful but that she feels awful and like a loser, the result is what is known as "blind-spot castration." (The word _castration_ may be a little harsh, as the condition is usually only temporary and men are able to recover from this feeling of impotence. We use the term here because men will know what we mean by it. Even if it seems like a sexist analogy, it is the word that has long been used to describe what many men experience when they feel as though they're losing with a woman.

We don't mean to imply that men can't be just as ugly or "bitchy" toward their partners. Men can attack women too, especially over their attractiveness, so this game of hurting one's partner is a two-way street.) Blind-spot castration is like a covert attack. The man feels like a loser but is confused about why he feels that way because he was just told how great he is. He did not see it coming, nor does he understand the dynamics of why he feels so poorly. A more direct sort of castration occurs when a woman tells a man he is a loser, a failure, and the cause of her misery. Although he still feels lousy, at least he understands why he is losing.

A woman can be miserable or in pain and not be doing it deliberately to hurt her man, yet he still will feel like he somehow failed. Vera and I have an ongoing argument about what kind of shoes she should wear when we take fairly long walks. I think high-heeled shoes look great and enhance a woman's appearance. When a woman does not have to walk a long way, heels are a fine choice of footwear. Vera is usually what I call sensible about this and wears a good walking shoe when we go on a long walk, but occasionally she will want to wear a shoe with high heels and little ankle support. I often catch her doing this before we leave the house, and she will usually change into something more comfortable. On a recent walk I did not notice until we were out the door that she was wearing a high-heeled shoe, and by the time I noticed she did not want to change them. We had fun on our walk and did not mention the shoes again. Later that evening I started to give her a foot massage, but she didn't want me to touch one foot because she had a painful blister there as a result of walking in those shoes. I felt like I had failed. She was in pain and I felt bad even though I knew that I had done everything reasonable to get her to wear the proper shoe. It did not matter that I saw it coming, could have predicted it, and understand this kind of stuff—I still felt blindsided.

Men and women who have been in a relationship for a long time sometimes play these sorts of funny games wherein one of them will act like the parent and the other like the child. Such dynamics can revolve around taking one's vitamins, eating properly, what to wear, flossing one's teeth, and countless other scenarios. The partners often will take turns in the role of parent and child. These games are just another way of relating and playing, and as long as they aren't the only way that the two relate to each other, we see no harm in playing them at times. This kind of behavior can be obnoxious to others, so it is probably better to only behave this way in private.

In the big scheme of things, a man's happiness does not depend exclusively on his woman's state of happiness or on her approval. There are many other factors involved, such as whether he is successful at work, whether his children are healthy, and his general mental health and well-being. That said, if all other factors are being met with winning results and his wife is unhappy, it will be difficult for him to be as happy as he would be otherwise.

∽ Insatiable Women ∽

We have met a few women who say that they want sex more often than their husbands or that they don't get it often enough from their lovers. We have found that these women were usually talking about intercourse rather than actual orgasm, because once their partners learned how to give them an EMO and they learned how to experience one, they no longer felt short-changed, and they stopped complaining about not getting enough. They wanted more intercourse because it wasn't totally fulfilling, yet it was enjoyable enough that they thought if they got more it would be more gratifying. A women's claim of sexual insatiability is also a way to cause her partner to feel inadequate and impotent; some of these women were using this strategy to beat up on their guys emotionally.

A man has to learn his craft as a student of the clitoris. He has to become confident in his knowledge of his partner's pleasure centers and his ability to take control of them. When a man learns to gratify his partner with his hands and possibly with his mouth, he will no longer have to feel impotent at any time. He will not have to rely on his penis to gratify her. He will be able to tell if she really wants more or is just saying so to support her claim of insatiability. Furthermore, he needs to know that waiting to have intercourse until after she has been orgasmic for an adequate amount of time makes the act of coitus that much more gratifying to a woman. As an added benefit, if the couple waits to start intercourse until well into the woman's orgasm, then the man won't have to worry about premature ejaculation because his partner will already have been coming for some time. The pressure will be off. A woman can admit honestly to wanting or not wanting to have intercourse, and her partner can know that he has given her great pleasure and satisfaction.

∽ Masturbation ∽

We have noticed that there are times when a woman wants to experience an orgasm but may not feel like reciprocating and playing with your penis, or she may feel like playing with your penis but for a shorter time than you would like. When this happens, instead of acting needy and pleading with her to continue, it is okay to finish yourself off with your own hand. It is also okay, of course, to ask her in a friendly way to get you off, but if she would prefer not to, you can do the job yourself. If both of you are in agreement and she is willing to lie there naked while you masturbate, it can be a lot of fun. Again, if she would prefer not to, you can do it in privacy. Every man we have met either masturbates frequently or has done so in his past. Some people still feel guilt over the act, but they do it anyway. We would like for people to think of masturbation as a wonderful and almost spiritual act. We recommend to many of our male clients that if they have to make any major decisions they should make sure that they get off first before deciding. They will be able to think more clearly, will have a much better perspective on any issue, and will therefore make much better choices.

∼ Getting to Be a Hero and Other Benefits ∼

It seems that men who are in a relationship with a woman live longer than their single brothers, but single women live just as long as married women. This indicates that, as far as relationships go, men probably require women more than women require men. As we have stated throughout this book, women are great at coming up with desires and goals in comparison with men. Men on their own will drive big pickup trucks with giant wheels. Some will fill their whole house with stereo equipment. If you see in the news that someone is riding across the country on a bicycle while sitting backwards, you can be certain that person is a man.

Women's goals are more wide-ranging and more pleasure-oriented than men's. A woman's goals will also include goals for the man she is with. Men on their own generally do only what they think they can accomplish. Women often have higher goals and aspirations for a man than he has for himself. He may doubt his ability to achieve a certain result, while she has only certainty. Her desire supplies a lot of energy, and when a man realizes this gift of vitality that comes with the request, it makes starting out on his quest that much easier. You do not have to doubt your ability, as you have the added power of her desire. And you must not doubt her attractiveness, as that, too, will short-circuit your action.

One becomes a hero by doing something that one believes is almost impossible to accomplish. Again, men on their own will not even attempt to do these kinds of things. To realize their potential they require someone outside of them—be it a boss, a coach, or best of all a woman—to have confidence in them. All of a sudden the impossible becomes possible, and they can do deeds that at one time seemed unattainable. That is the road of the hero. A man must realize that he has extra power because he has a woman's desires fanning the flames, as Mama Gena likes to say, of his engine. He will do well to think of his abilities as expanded, as long as he is filling those desires.

A woman will usually not surrender to a man until she feels that he has surrendered to her. She wants the man to say yes to her wants and desires before she says yes to his. A woman often holds out, especially in the area of pleasure, until she is sure that the man is fun and is deserving of her. Willingness is an extremely important attitude for a man to have, both in the beginning of a relationship and after years of marriage. The fact that he would be willing to say yes to almost anything that his woman wants puts him in a place of appreciation and will make his life more pleasant. Because he is willing to say yes, most women will tend to ask only for things they have a real desire for. When a man holds out in some area, whether it be money, time, or sexual attention, it seems to create a state wherein the woman wants whatever he is withholding from her. A man who says yes to a woman's wants either will be able to produce those desires easily or will find that she no longer wants them. In either case he will be ahead in the game. The man who says no will have an unhappy woman on his hands and will probably wind up doing what he originally said no to anyway. It is more fun to do things for your woman enthusiastically than to do them kicking and screaming.

We knew a couple who were married for a few years when the wife decided that she wanted a house and also wanted to go back to college. Her husband complained to us that they could not afford one of the things, let alone both of them, and it was driving him crazy. We told him just to say yes, not necessarily even to do anything, but just to say okay. He took our advice and a few months later they found a house for a reasonable price. His wife started to go to school at nights and still kept her day job. She graduated about five years later and at that point they sold their house for over a hundred thousand dollars in profit. They were able to buy an even better home and she was able to get a better-paying job, just because he had said yes.

∾ Romance ∾

Once people get married they often seem to change toward each other and to lose some of the fun in their relationship. This is where good communication skills are important to keep the relationship fresh. People often start taking one another for granted and forget how to be nice to one another. A shortage of acknowledging can set in that can result in feelings of being unappreciated, or worse. By staying up-to-date in your communication, especially noticing and appreciating good things about one another whenever you can, you will stay ahead of the marriage demons and continue to have fun together.

Another way a man can show his love is by being romantic. Continue to romance the woman you married as if you were still courting her. Having a woman whom you love in your life provides a wonderful opportunity to open up your barrel of love. By doing romantic things for her you are really doing them for yourself. You are the one who can get the most out of being romantic. It is a side of humanity that many men have been conditioned not to experience, yet it can be a powerful and wonderful feeling to be able to express your love and devotion. You do not have to spend a whole lot of money to be romantic. Vera says that women give out points for each nice thing a guy does for them, and you only get one point no matter how big or expensive the deed is, and it has to be given unconditionally and with love. Flowers, poetry, chocolates, pretty cards with sweet words written on them—all are fun to do and will get you points, although you must not do it for the points.

Sometimes men do something romantic because they have hurt their partner or because they feel guilty over some indiscretion. George Burns told a cute story about flirting with some woman, and because he felt guilty, he bought Gracie a beautiful silver centerpiece. Neither of them mentioned his transgression. Ten years later George overheard Gracie saying to one of her friends that she wished George would flirt with another woman because she could use another centerpiece.

When a man romances a woman without expecting anything in return it can open a woman's sexual barrel, which she, in turn, has been conditioned to keep a lid on. A woman who is romanced is more likely to unleash her sexual, animalistic side and to show some real appetite for orgasmic pleasures. If a woman does unleash her sexual nature, it actually causes the man to feel even more romantic and to romance her more often. More romance activates more fun in bed, which instigates more romance. It can be a lovely cycle to travel.

⌒ Not to Bed? ⌒

As we wrote in Chapter 6, "Her Side of the Bed," it is the woman's vote that ultimately decides when and if there will be any going to bed, as the man's vote is almost always yes. A woman wants her man to want to go to bed with her, because his saying yes is proof of her attractiveness. For this reason, it is usually a good idea to make attractive offers to a woman to show her that you are interested. As long as you are not pestering or nagging her constantly, she will appreciate the offers, though not always with an acceptance. Unless it is a matter of either party's religious beliefs, a woman will think that a man who does not want to go to bed with her may have something wrong with him or may be gay. If they have been together for a number of years, she may think he is cheating on her. As we've said, a man must follow his integrity about whether or not to go to bed. When he does vote no, to avoid misunderstandings, it can be a good idea to let her know why. There are some valid reasons not to go to bed. Maybe he has a sense that there is no real desire on her part and she is only doing it because she thinks she should, or maybe he has an injury he hasn't told her about, or perhaps he is just too tired. When there is real desire and turn-on coming from a woman it is amazing how a man can forget that he is tired and start to feel energetic. If she cannot seduce him from being too tired, he can promise to take care of her the next morning.

Sometimes a man will say no to going to bed because he has lost in bed too many times in the past. Since men want to win more than anything else, the idea of going to a place associated with losing will make a man want to stay away. The next chapter, "Under the Covers: All You Both Need to Know for Great Sex," outlines communication skills for both men and women that, if practiced, will guarantee a winning time in bed. It also offers more insight into how to give your partner lots of pleasure in bed—from basic attitudes you can embrace to specific techniques you can employ.

✧ EXERCISE 7 ✧
Self-Pleasure for Men

Most men have at one time or another masturbated, probably on a somewhat regular basis. Men usually "jerk off" or "spank the monkey," as it is sometimes called, to relieve themselves of sexual tension or tumescence. They accomplish the act by tensing up, rubbing themselves hard and fast, and trying to ejaculate as quickly as possible. By contrast, in this exercise the only goal is to do it sensually, which means to touch yourself just for the good sensation you are feeling at the moment with no ejaculatory goals in the future.

It can be a good idea to set up your space as you did for the "visiting dignitary" exercise in Chapter 1. Use whatever aids you like that help you feel aroused, such as a sexy magazine, a pornography video, or a fantasy. Do the exercise in a comfortable space, such as your bed, rather than over the toilet. Make sure no one will disturb you. Turn the phone ringer off and close the door if you live with someone else. Let your partner, roommate, or family members know that you are not to be interrupted unless there is some dire emergency.

Begin by touching yourself lightly around your genitals, in a teasing fashion. When you're ready, put some lubricant, such as Vaseline or Albolene or a water-soluble kind, on your hand and lubricate your penis. There is no exact or best way to do this; we recommend experimenting by doing it a different way every time to find out how you like it best. You can take your time and touch a small part of your penis with the lubricant, or do it more quickly and cover the whole penis. Just make sure you are enjoying every touch and stroke. It is not even necessary to have a hard penis; just enjoy the touch. Make sure your pubic hair is out of the way, including loose hairs. Once you're lubricated, start stroking yourself in a rhythmical, steady way that feels pleasurable.

Usually when the same stroke is used repeatedly it feels better and better. If at any time you feel like switching or taking a break, it is okay to do so. Relax as much as possible, as you will be able to feel more that way than if you're tensed up (which is how most men usually masturbate).

When you're ready, try peaking. Peaking is the deliberate creation of a high point in the amount of sensation you're experiencing. Do this by changing or stopping the stroking before the sensation dissipates on its own. By changing the stroke, which you can accomplish by changing either the pressure, the location, or the speed, or by stopping altogether, you will feel less sensation, thereby creating a peak. Then, when you start stroking again in a deliberate, steady, reliable way, the sensation will rise. Each peak is a complete cycle; you can create as many peaks or cycles as you want. When you deliberately bring the sensation down, it allows you to go up again on the next peak. By contrast, if you were to keep rubbing, you would either go numb or begin to ejaculate.

We recommend to our students to get as close to ejaculation as they can without going over—that is, to peak themselves right before ejaculation. Some clear fluid may be released from your penis, but see if you can stop before the ejaculation begins. A good way to keep from ejaculating is to press firmly under the scrotum (the location of the ejaculatory duct) for a couple of seconds. Another way is to take your hand off your penis right before you start squirting. A third way is to firmly squeeze the head of your penis. Now start stroking again. After each peak or cycle you can experiment with a different kind of stroke, or you can keep doing each cycle with the same stroke. The goal is to experiment, have fun, and experience as much sensation as you can.

Peak yourself as many times as feels good to you. If you find yourself unable to put off ejaculation any longer, keep stroking through the ejaculation, using progressively lighter strokes, and perhaps experimenting with using slower stokes, too. The goal of this exercise is not to ejaculate, although doing so is okay. The goal is to feel as much as you can, to relax, to experiment with different kinds of strokes, to build up as much sensation as you can, and to enjoy every moment of the activity. As we stated, it is okay not to have an engorged penis while doing this exercise. Just enjoy the touch; a flaccid penis can feel a lot of pleasure, too. Do not put pressure on yourself in any way that feels stressful. If after doing this exercise you still have sexual tension, by all means spank your monkey.

By learning what feels best and most pleasurable, you will be able to teach your partner how and where you prefer to be touched. By learning the technique of peaking you will be able to use this understanding to improve your ability to do it to your partner. The idea is the same whether the pleasure recipient is a male or a female: to stop right before they have had enough so that you can extend their pleasure further.

∼ Chapter Highlights

♦ Penises don't lie!

♦ It is really a lack of communication between the man and the woman that leads to the lack or loss of engorgement.

♦ The most important kind of communication you can engage in while in bed is to report all the wonderful feelings and sensations you're experiencing and also the ones you notice in your partner.

♦ The clitoris is a slippery little organ. It will dive into the body, hide under the hood, and avoid intimacy until you prove your skills at wooing it into surrender.

♦ Most women like a lighter touch than most men.

♦ When a man learns to gratify a woman with his hands and possibly also with his mouth, he will no longer have to feel impotent at any time.

CHAPTER 8

I will follow you,
my dear,

Till ever allows and
more.

I shall treasure each
moment where

We share each
other's core.

Under the Covers

All You Both Need to Know for Great Sex

*H*aving decided to go to bed, it is now time to go under the covers. By "going under the covers" we mean creating the most fun possible in bed. In this chapter we describe some of the fundamental techniques for taking control of your partner's nervous system, including trusting your feelings, being curious, enjoying yourself at all times, and focusing your attention and intention.

We have spent a large part of this book emphasizing the importance of the clitoris, but before getting to the clitoris a man has to learn about women and especially about the specific woman he is with. Many men are uninformed when it comes to women. Women do not always reveal themselves, and men are not inclined to ask. In earlier chapters we described some of the things and experiences that women want. Women's bodies are very pleasure-oriented, but a man must know how to explore them and how to get a woman to want to be explored and stimulated. Women can learn to teach men more about their bodies and about how they like to be touched, and they can also learn more about men's bodies and how to touch them. So in order to get under the covers you first have to remove some of the covers separating yourself from your partner. Helping you do this is the primary aim of this whole book.

∾ Men's Resistance in Bed ∾

The same techniques used to seduce someone to get into bed can be used to continue to seduce them once you are under the covers. Seduction at this level takes lots of attention and offers an opportunity to have lots of fun. A woman may still resist a man's advances and good intentions even after she has gotten naked and appears to be ready for intense pleasure. Earlier chapters address in detail how to deal with a woman's resistance to pleasure. By contrast, a man who has gotten naked and is already under the covers has usually given up most of his resistances; at this stage any move on the woman's part to seduce and stimulate him can bear results quite easily.

The only resistance some men may have at this point is a resistance to letting the woman have her way with him. A man may want to stay in control and may find the prospect of surrendering that control a bit scary. But he has already decided to have some pleasure, so he can most likely be convinced to let go with a little urging. He may try to stay in control and dictate what his lover is doing to him, but he can be easily persuaded to surrender by a confident woman. A woman who wants to give her man pleasure has to take control of his body just as he must learn how to take control of her body. The difference is that a woman can engorge a man without touching him; she can do it with just her desire. She can turn him into her sex object simply by wanting to. When a woman really wants to give a man pleasure there is little he can say or do to resist her. Vera does not have to ask me if she can touch me and give me an orgasm. She does not have to seduce me with words or tricks of any kind. All she has to do is start and I'm putty in her hands or mouth. Actually, when Vera asks me if she can rub on my penis, it almost feels like the right answer is no, because she does not have to ask; all she has to do is start touching me. As we stated earlier, an engorged penis is bisexually owned, meaning that when she gets me hard, she is as much the rightful owner of that penis as I am, and she can do to it whatever she wants in the name of enjoyment.

∿ How to Avoid Making Your Partner Gag ∿

When a woman finally admits to wanting some orgasmic pleasure, the game is not over. At that point a man must continue to play. He must notice when it is time to go for the intense orgasm, when it is time to tease and hold back, when it is time to take a break, and when it is time to stop. This means he must continue to pay attention to her so he can tell which way she is going: toward him or away, up or down, filled up or still empty.

Many men have a tendency to overproduce, to keep giving a woman things or experiences till she is gagging. When you look at your partner and notice that she is blue in the face and not breathing, you know that you have gone too far. When a man finds something his woman likes, whether it be ice cream, fellatio, cunnilingus, or even an EMO, he will be inclined to continue presenting her with it until she starts throwing up, so to speak, which is evidenced by her being no longer thrilled (and probably annoyed) at his behavior. By focusing his attention on her he can notice when this change occurs and can learn to stop even sooner next time. When Vera told me how much she liked a specific brand of bran muffin, I purchased them practically every day until our refrigerator and freezer were full of them. We would open the freezer door and the muffins would tumble out. I did not give her an adequate amount of time to swallow and appreciate them. Because I overproduced on the muffin front, she got sick of them and we wound up throwing most of them out or giving them away.

The same thing can happen sexually. For example, when a man learns how to give a woman an extended massive orgasm, he sometimes becomes overzealous in this pursuit and wants to rub on her for an hour or more at a time. Although Vera and I do demonstrations that are an hour long to show what is humanly possible, it is not something we do all the time and definitely not something we recommend for someone who is new to this possibility. More than one student has told us that after they and their partner had an hour-long (or longer) EMO they did not want to do it again for quite a while. This is because they were doing it as a matter of production instead of for the sheer pleasure of doing it. Rather, we encourage our students to enjoy the exquisite sensation of a few strokes on the right place at the right time, and then to back off and allow the pleasure recipient to swallow the experience.

We have had a number of women students who had never before experienced an orgasm. They are like a person who has not eaten in a long time. They see food and they want to eat it all, but their stomachs are shrunk so they can only ingest a small amount. When their lovers learn how to gratify them, they want to give these women more than they can consume. This means the man is not paying attention to his partner. Notice her response to each stroke and you will be able to tell when to continue and when to stop. Remember, too, that many women who are new to the technique of relaxing while being stimulated miss the rush they have always associated with orgasm. The two of you can agree ahead of time that at the end of the experience the woman can tense up and go over the edge if she likes. Just make sure she knows it is deliberate on your part. After practicing the relaxed type of orgasm most women will learn that they can have even more fun and greater pleasure without tensing up at the end.

Here's a side note on the literal (as opposed to the metaphorical) topic of gagging: There is a sexual act called "throat fucking," wherein the woman lies passively, usually on a bed with her head hanging over the side. The man straddles her face and she allows him to insert his erect penis into her mouth and to thrust deeply, as if he were performing intercourse. We have known only a few women who enjoy this activity. The woman must be very relaxed and trusting; otherwise her gag reflex will be activated, which isn't very pleasurable. The act can be quite erotic but is generally better to watch on a porno tape than to actually do.

∼ Choosing to Be a Pleasure Victim ∼

Being a victim is either a role that one can don in certain circumstances or a persona that one can adopt for most of his or her life. Playing the victim can be the best choice in certain circumstances in order to obtain one's goals or to get one's ideas across; for example, when you've been stopped by the police for a traffic violation or when a child needs to gain attention from his or her parents because she is sick and needs assistance. Sometimes when people act as if they are unable to function without help, they receive beneficial aid or win money in a lawsuit. And choosing to be a victim of pleasure can cause a person to maximize his or her enjoyment during a sensual experience. So playing the victim's role can be a good choice once in a while. However, if a person habitually chooses to be the victim, he or she will frequently be out of agreement with his or her life and will generally be unhappy. Habitual victims do, in fact, have a choice about whether or not to play the victim, but because they've become almost addicted to losing and being unhappy, they refuse to admit or see their own responsibility for their situation. There is a difference between playing the victim when it serves you and feeling like a victim by default.

As we mentioned above and touched on in Chapter 2, it can prove beneficial and highly erotic to be a pleasure victim, the one who gives up control, the recipient of someone else's total attention. However, surrendering sexually to another person for pleasure purposes is difficult to do in our society. Everyone wants to be in control, and to surrender your nervous system to someone else makes you very vulnerable and is very scary. Pardon the vulgarity, but in our culture it is okay to fuck someone, but to *be* fucked or *get* fucked is a metaphor for being a loser. Fucking is actually something that you do *with* someone, but the way we use the word makes it seem like either you are doing it *to* someone or someone is doing it to you. It is difficult to surrender while fucking, and it takes both parties being actively involved to create the best fucks. On the other hand, if we remove intercourse (that is, fucking) from the equation, it may be easier to give up control to another person if he or she is stimulating your body, specifically your genitals, with his or her hands and/or mouth.

To play the game of pleasure victim, one person takes the control seat and the other person surrenders. As we have mentioned, this divvying up of roles creates an opportunity for the highest level of orgasm and the most intense sensations. The one who surrenders, or the pleasure victim, remains totally "at effect" (that is, receives attention without giving any in return) during the experience. The one in control can do whatever he or she wants to do to make his or her victim feel blissful and ecstatic, within the agreed-upon limits that the two parties previously established, either verbally or nonverbally. All the pleasure victim has to do is lie there and feel gratified and wonderful. It helps for the victim to verbally acknowledge all the wonderful sensations he or she is feeling, but not to the point where doing so interferes with his or her pleasure, as can happen if a person talks too much or moans too loudly or tries too hard to impress the other. Verbal acknowledgment and appreciation are of utmost significance, because as we described earlier, the third ingredient of a gratified appetite is verbal appreciation while the sensual interlude is occurring and verbal acknowledgment of the shared fun afterward.

The more trust and confidence a person has in their own abilities to be pleasured, the easier it is for them to assume the role of the pleasure victim or to surrender. Vera, who has trained for many years to have EMOs and to feel tremendous amounts of pleasurable sensations in her body, is able to allow herself to be pleasurably touched and stimulated by any student who happens to be learning how to produce pleasure. The more a person trains his or her own body to receive intense pleasure, the easier it becomes for him or her to be able to surrender to anyone. The more doubt someone has about his or her ability to receive sensual pleasure, the harder it is for that person to surrender his or her nervous system to anyone.

It is also true that the more confidence and trust someone has in the abilities of the person who will be taking control, the more of themselves they will surrender. Therefore, if a person wants their partner to surrender and to become their pleasure victim, they will have to demonstrate confidence, self-assurance, and integrity. They will have to show their partner that they know and enjoy what they are doing, they will have to be playful and tease the victim mercilessly, they will have to be curious and have fun, and they will have to demonstrate high levels of intention and attention. (We will describe each of these attributes in more detail shortly.)

All these ingredients combined allow a person to surrender and let you take them for a ride. If you demonstrate these attributes, you will inspire confidence in your partner that the purpose of the game is to give them great pleasure. It is to make their capacity for pleasure (if there is a capacity) extend to its outermost limits. The only way a person can reach those outer limits is by surrendering totally, and the only way they can surrender totally is if the person they are surrendering to is trained and highly motivated to demonstrate his or her ability and desire to take control of the "victim's" nervous system at the appropriate time.

∿ Know What You Are Doing ∿

This all means that one has to learn one's craft in order to be the best lover that anyone would want to have. It means doing it the same way you've always done it—including neglecting to learn how to communicate, and failing to learn how to touch your partner exactly how they like to be touched—will no longer be an option. Once you know that something better is available and once you've learned how to obtain it, better becomes the only option. Mediocrity is simply no longer viable. Even though you don't have a choice in the matter, this is good news for you and your partner, because the result is more fun and a better sex life. A better sex life starts with one that is good now, yet is enhanced by your belief that it will improve in the future.

Every person has preferences about how they like to be touched. Some people like light pressure, some like it more vigorous. Some like to hear their lovers talk nasty, others prefer only sweet words. Everyone has erogenous zones, but not everyone has the same erogenous zones. Different areas of the body will yield results that are more or less sensational depending on who is doing the touching, whom one is touching, how one is doing the touching, and which areas are most sensitive. However, the thing everyone has in common is that the more a person is able to surrender and relax his or her body, the greater the variety of touches that will produce wonderfully pleasurable sensations.

A person can only reach a limited level of confidence from reading a book. It is the actual practicing of the techniques with your partner that will take you to the next level in your skills in bed. Meanwhile, pretend and act as confident as you can without being belligerent. It is usually best to be polite and kind. Never get pissed at your partner for behaving in a way contrary to what you want. Instead, seduce him or her into behavior that makes both of you feel good. Remember that resistances are not bad; they are just obstacles that, once overcome, will make the whole experience more valuable and more fun. The conquering of resistances adds power to the equation that can be exploited and turned into orgasmic energy. As practitioners of the martial arts do, use your partner's resistance to create more energy and thus more pleasure for both of you.

∾ Trust Your Feelings ∾

It is important when making love to trust your feelings. Your feelings will not lie to you, and if you can trust them and express them to your partner in a respectful and kind way, you will raise your sexual expertise to a higher level. When we are in intimate relationships, and especially when we are in the midst of a sensual experience, we all have thoughts pop into our minds about what's going in at any given moment. These are not just energy waves that your brain is playing with. Each thought has some meaning to you, and by glossing it over, refusing to pay attention to it, or discounting it as stupid or silly, you hamper your abilities as a lover. Maybe a thought flits through your head that says, "What she just said to me did not feel friendly," or "The last couple of strokes he made weren't as gratifying as the previous ones," or "Why is she touching me like this?" These and a million other thoughts will crop up in your life, not just your sex life, and addressing them by verbally communicating them to your partner in a civil and friendly manner enables the intimacy between the two of you to evolve.

This is related to the topic of integrity, which we addressed in Chapter 5. If your partner is carrying on, moaning wildly, acting like they are in the throes of a fantastic orgasm, yet you sense on some level that they may be pretending, you are probably right. Take a break and check in with your partner. Tell them you sense a discrepancy between how they are acting and what you are feeling. Let them know you are there for them but you do not want "faked" pleasure. Tell them you want them to feel true pleasure and intense sensations, and that you can tell the difference between real and imaginary feelings. Communicate all this in a kind and lighthearted way so your partner doesn't get angry and totally withdraw.

We have had clients who would moan loudly, even if the sensation in their genitals was only minimal. Since we were the teachers, we could tell them they were not allowed to moan at all until we said they could. We told them we felt some sensation in their clitoris, but compared to how much they were carrying on, it was negligible. We asked them how they thought they would sound when they really started feeling more. They knew that we knew what we were doing, and they knew that they could not easily pull the wool over our eyes. Our telling them this actually helped them to surrender more. Since you and are partner do not hold the positions of teacher and student, it is still important that you speak up when you sense some discrepancy, but remember to do it in such a way so as not to create any anger. It is always a good idea to ask questions, for example, "Do you think the intensity of your orgasm is equal to your moans?" When you catch your partner exaggerating in this way, he or she will respect you and will surrender to you even more next time you take control. Sometimes a person's wild sounds do equal the sensation they are feeling. When that's the case, the loud joyful growling won't distract or divert your attention away from the pleasure at hand. In fact, it can add to the awesome positive experience of orgasmic bliss.

It is good to speak up whenever something is going on that feels funny or strange to you or that causes you to wonder or your thoughts to wander. A woman was rubbing on me one time, and it felt good, but she kept switching strokes, so it seemed like she did not know what she was doing. As a result I found it difficult to surrender. I told her how I was feeling, and she responded that she was doing it deliberately because she wanted to keep me going for a longer time than usual. Once I understood what she was doing and that it was on purpose, I could surrender more easily and allow her to do her thing to me without my wondering if she knew what she was up to. If I had not spoken up, the teasing would have continued to feel like a sort of torture. However, it would have been even better had she told me from the beginning what she was doing and then kept me updated the whole time she was stroking me.

Sometimes you can be rubbing and stimulating your pleasure victim and everything seems to be going well, and all of a sudden you sense a change. It no longer feels as good and you detect that something may be wrong—yet no one is talking. This is a perfect time to take a break and check in with your partner. What you're picking up on could be caused by any number of things. Maybe a loose pubic hair has found its way under your finger and is irritating your partner's skin. In any case it is time to peak your partner and to bring them down a bit before you continue with any stimulation that will take them higher. Remember that what you feel and notice are valid, and the only way you can become an accomplished lover is to trust your feelings and thoughts.

∾ Enjoy What You Are Doing ∾

The only way your partner—man or woman—can reap the most fun from being your pleasure victim is if you are thoroughly enjoying producing pleasure with him or her. This means every time you touch your partner, every time you kiss your partner, and every moment you spend seducing your partner, you must do so for strictly selfish motives because you get gratification from it. To do otherwise will create a feeling that you are owed something, and nobody wants to surrender if they sense that you are just pleasuring them in order to get something later. Even the best prostitutes are the ones who take the most enjoyment from giving another person pleasure.

Most of you are not prostitutes. You are not getting paid for having to give someone else fun. If you cannot take enjoyment from giving someone touches and attention, then you have no business being in that situation. Just because you created a wonderful opportunity for your partner to surrender and become a pleasure victim does not mean your partner has to return the favor and do the same for you. They can reciprocate if they want to, either immediately afterward or later, but they are not required to rub your back just because you rubbed theirs. By rubbing theirs you got yours, and to insist otherwise only throws sand into the machinery.

How can you derive the most pleasure possible from the sensual experience you are creating for your partner? Take delight in each breath she produces, each sound emanating from him, each touch of her skin, each word he utters. Smell the wonderful scent of her pleasure; observe the wondrous glistening of his blissful body caught up in your magnificent creation. Heighten her experience with a fantasy that energizes her and that you enjoy making up. Tease him to the point where he is begging for more. Report any feelings, sensations, and signs of pleasure that you notice in your partner or in yourself, as well as any positive thoughts you're having. The more one appreciates something the better it becomes. Encourage your partner to also report any pleasurable sensations he or she experiences. By first doing so yourself, you in essence create a space for your partner to do the same.

∼ Be Playful and Curious ∼

Playfulness and curiosity are important attributes to add to your toolbox if you want to produce the most delight for yourself and your partner. When we suggest being playful, we mean be ready to respond to any and all kinds of resistance with a lighthearted attitude and a sense of humor. It can be useful to stay one step ahead of your pleasure victim by anticipating where they may resist and throwing them a curveball when they expected a fastball down the center of the plate. This will keep them off balance enough to prevent them from predicting with certainty what your next move will be. On one hand, it is important to be predictable, to use a steady and rhythmic stroke when touching your lover's erogenous zones. This allows your partner to feel safe and to relax into the next stroke with some dependability. On the other hand, if your lover can too easily predict what you will be doing next, he or she may tend to resist what is coming or may go unconscious. There's a fine line here, and you have to learn which side to deliver from. It depends on your partner's resistance, on his or her particular mood that day, and on how well she or he can relax under different circumstances. Remember from Chapter 2 how we talked about there being several categories of pleasure victims and of seducers? No one fits into a single category at all times. Sometimes the reliable, predictable, and honorable way is the best path into your lover's heart, and at other times displaying your rascally, unpredictable, unreliable side works best. This is what we mean by being playful: Be ready to do and be whatever and whoever it takes to get the best results.

By going with what feels right at the time—by using the integrity we've written about—you will notice that each sensual episode will play out in different ways. Sometimes you will feel like teasing your partner till they cannot take it anymore, and at other times you will sense that the best thing to do is to go directly for their most sensitive spot without delay. This is where curiosity comes in. Experiment with new and different styles and techniques each time out. Go to the bookstore and find new sex books that you can read for yourself or share with your partner. The more open and willing you are to explore each time you have a sexual experience, the more fun it will be for you. If you like, keep a journal of all the different skills and techniques you have tried.

When you are giving your partner pleasure it can be helpful to find out what they are feeling, what they like, and what they would prefer. It is best to ask them easy questions that don't require much thought to answer. As we described in the exercises at the end of Chapter 5, asking yes-or-no questions is best. Good questions include ones like "Would you like more pressure?" "Would you prefer less pressure?" "Do you want me to move my touch more to the left?" "... more to the right?" "... higher?" "... lower?" "... deeper under the hood?" Ask whatever seems appropriate and reasonable. This is one aspect of being curious: showing interest in what your partner likes. As we also described in the Chapter 5 exercises, avoid questions like "Do you like this?" or "Does this feel good?" because your partner may want to avoid hurting your feelings and so may lie rather than risk doing so.

After the sensual interlude is over it can help to go over the experience with your partner, to find out if there was something different or extra you could have done to make it even better. You can also use this postmortem discussion to tell your partner about specific moments you really enjoyed. We call this form of feedback "giving specific frames," just as a frame in a motion picture equals one frozen moment in an ongoing movie. Noticing and talking about specific wonderful moments will add to the experience and enable you and your lover to go higher. When you think and communicate in terms of specific frames, you feel like you are reliving the moment. For example, if you were to describe to a third party a specific frame from a sensual interlude you created with your lover, that person could potentially feel the turn-on and the positive charge from the episode. If, on the other hand, you were to tell them about the experience without using specific frames, it would seem duller and less interesting. Note that at first it can be challenging to remember specific moments. It really helps to remember them afterward if you first report them in real time, that is, during the experience itself. Doing so will both enhance the experience and enable you to remember the moment later when you are reliving it with your lover.

Another benefit of having a playful attitude is that it helps you avoid getting upset when your partner says or does anything mean or negative. You will be able to respond to what they say and do without getting ugly in return. Their negativity is just another form of resistance, and your best response may be to back off more than they really wanted or expected you to. It is the same as the game of seduction: When your target is coming toward you, you can fill them with as much as they can handle, but when they show the first signs of resistance or pulling away, you have to back away even further, to the point of being willing to end the experience entirely. This is where paying attention is so important, because you must be able to notice whether someone is coming toward you or going away from you.

∽ Attention ∽

Exercising one's integrity is very important in the game of love, but if one lacks the ability to pay attention to what he or she is doing, one will miss many of the signals that would help him or her know how to do so. When you are first learning how to give an EMO or how to be the pleasure meister to your pleasure victim, it may be a good idea to go for only short periods of time so you can build up your ability to stay attentive and focused for longer periods of time. Engage in these acts a little longer each time out. It is like lifting weights: You wouldn't try to bench press an excessive amount of weight the first time; rather, you would gradually increase the weight at each session till you were able to lift successively heavier amounts. How long you go will also depend on how much attention your partner is able to take. People who are not used to a lot of attention may be unable to just lie there and relax and be at effect for long periods of time when they are first introduced to the ways of the pleasure victim. This is where your attention is so vital: You must notice when they've received enough and then learn to back off before this happens. This is what peaking is about. If you peak your partner *before* he or she has had enough, you will be able to start again a lot sooner than if you had waited until your partner had to inform you that he or she had received a sufficient amount of stimulation.

Even while your attention is on your partner, you also have to notice the feelings in your own body, especially in the fingers and hands you're using to touch your partner. You must be aware of all the signs of pleasure that your partner is showing and also be conscious of whether the pleasure in your own body is waxing or waning. These changes in levels of pleasurable sensation can be quite minute and therefore require your full attention at all times. When a person goes unconscious for a few seconds and misses some strokes or fails to notice that their pleasure victim has also gone unconscious, they will lose control; their partner cannot surrender to an unconscious person. It is quite common for both the victim of pleasure and the giver of pleasure to go unconscious at the same time. This is why it is so important to stay conscious and to have your full attention trained on your partner at all times, because when the pleasure victim goes unconscious, it is already past time for a break.

Keeping your attention focused is helped by reporting any signs of pleasure and orgasm that your partner is demonstrating and also by reporting how his or her response makes you feel. This ongoing verbalization also helps your partner sense your attention and, thus, to surrender to what you are doing. She or he won't be surprised by anything you happen to be doing, which enables her or him to relax more while under your control. Surprises naturally bring people down. If this is what you intend to do, then it is okay, but if it is not your intention to bring your partner down, then do not employ surprises. By verbalizing almost constantly when you are the one in control, you will stay in present time, focused on what you are doing. You will be unable to slip into your head and allow your thoughts to wander off to somewhere else. Your attention will remain focused on pleasure and on your pleasure victim.

⌇ Intention ⌇

In the preceding paragraph we mentioned the use of intention. One of Dr. Victor Baranco's favorite lines is "True intention is demonstrated by attainment." This means that by looking at the final results, you can tell if a person really had the aim they started out with, or if they were just doing something halfheartedly and without genuine purpose. Sexually speaking, if one wants to take his or her partner higher but the partner goes down, then he or she did not hold the full intention that would have gotten the partner to the desired destination. The same is true if you want to bring your partner down but instead the partner goes up. The manifestation—the end result—shows that you lacked true intention. Once you notice that your intentions have not manifested, it is best to get into agreement with the way things are going. Doing so will allow you to regain control. As long as your intentions and the outcome are at odds, you will remain out of control. Trying is the opposite of intention. When somebody tries to raise their hand, they fail. Trying means failing and intending means attaining.

When creating a space and a time for someone to be your pleasure victim, the power of your intention will prove important if your intended victim is going to give it up to you and surrender his or her nervous system. If you approach the experience halfheartedly, your partner will feel your apathy as a lack of intention. A person can also feel when you are thoroughly engaged in the process of their pleasure. This makes their decision to surrender that much easier. By holding true intention you remain focused on the goal, which is pleasure at all times.

Holding real intention is at least as important as what you are actually doing to your partner. It is the intention behind the stroke that determines whether your partner goes up or down in sensation. The same stroke with opposite intention will cause an opposite effect. For example, the use of a firmer pressure is normally associated with bringing someone down, but if one intends to use firm pressure to take someone higher, it can be an effective technique for doing so.

Your actions will have their best effect on your pleasure victim if they seem to be done on purpose rather than haphazardly. If you notice that your finger has moved from the spot where it was, or if you momentarily slip into a state of less awareness than you had planned, get into accord with what has happened and claim it as part of your intended action. Own that it did not occur by accident but on purpose. If you are rubbing on a woman's clitoris and you notice that all of a sudden your finger is on top of her hood, quickly take responsibility for where you are. Let her know that you're rubbing on her hood and that you will get back to the clitoris when you feel she can handle more. This way, you stay in control, and you and your intention are back on the same page.

Your attention keeps your intention focused, which allows true attainment of pleasure every step of the way. This goes for both women and men who wish to gain the confidence and trust of their partners in order to coax them into surrender.

∼ Two-Way Pleasure ∼

We've talked quite a bit in this chapter about active and passive parties to pleasure, but pleasure doesn't always have to be one-sided. It can be fun to lie in bed with your partner while both of you touch and tease and probe and kiss and fondle each other. This certainly isn't bad, and it is how most people make love. We present the one-sided technique as something new to add to whatever you are already doing. It also happens to be the optimum way for creating the highest orgasmic response in a person. A fantastic, high-level orgasm may or may not be what a couple wants each time they go to bed. They may want to hold each other in their arms and wrap their legs around each other and squeeze and cuddle each other. This sounds like intercourse, but penetration doesn't have to occur with every squeeze between two naked bodies. Of course, intercourse is still an option that a couple can choose when both partners want it. Intercourse is best when both parties actively take and give as much pleasure as they can.

There are dozens of intercourse positions—just read the *Kama Sutra*—and to be enjoyable, most if not all of them require the full action and response of both people. A woman may sometimes have intercourse because she thinks she should, because she thinks it is what everyone does, or just to get her man off her back by squirting him with her vagina and her pelvis. If a man wants to be a good lover he must first learn how to rub on his partner's clitoris and genitals, and he must learn to notice if she really wants to have intercourse or is just doing it as a service for him. A man can learn with practice and dedication and attention how to be a great lover and how to tell whether his partner is faking it, just going through the motions, or really wanting it.

If a woman doesn't really want intercourse, an experienced and attentive partner will be able to notice this and will be certain not to engage in any penetration. The fun to be had during intercourse, when the woman totally desires it, is so much more pleasurable than the alternative that it will become an easy choice to make even though the frequency of intercourse may go down. I cannot remember the last time Vera and I had intercourse without my first playing with her clitoris. Doing it the other way just does not make sense, because when I first stimulate her, our lovemaking becomes both more fun for me and definitely more pleasurable for her. Nor do I rub her clitoris for the primary purpose of making her eager for penile penetration. I rub her clitoris as an act in itself. It does not have to lead anywhere. Now more than ever, it often seems that after I've stimulated her genitals for a while, perhaps twenty minutes, she really wants my penis and will either take it in her hands or mouth or, rather frequently, will want vaginal penetration. She almost always uses some form of lubricant on my penis when rubbing it and makes sure it is lubricated before penetration. Some women are really wet, making lubrication unnecessary before insertion, but as women get older they have less natural lubrication. In that case it is important to use lubricant to ensure that penetration is neither difficult nor painful to either party. We think using lubricant makes things feel better and adds to the experience. We encourage you not to feel any shame about using it.

Our favorite position for intercourse is what we call the "conversational position." We lie on the bed, side-by-side. I am usually on Vera's right. I lie on my left side facing her, and she lies on her right side facing me. We bring our bodies close together, especially at our pelvises, and intertwine our legs. My penis can easily slip into her vagina from underneath and behind, or she can guide it in with her hand. Because we're facing each other, we can talk while we are engaged or she can move her body in an almost spooning position. We can also reposition our legs, unwrapping them and rewrapping them together in various configurations, and rubbing them against one another's. No matter what position you're using, you and your partner can move your pelvises in, out, up, and down to achieve maximum sensation during intercourse.

∾ Slooowww Down ∾

We think many people go way too fast when they're having intercourse. Moving slowly is recommended when you want to feel as much sensation as possible. This applies both to intercourse and to manual stimulation of the penis, even though many men are conditioned to liking it hard and fast. If you do it fast, like rabbits do it, you will miss much of the stroke. This might be okay sometimes, but for maximum pleasure you want to make your in-and-out movements slow. This way, you can feel the entire stroke and stay more relaxed, both of which are necessary for getting the most pleasure and sensation possible.

We recommend the slooowww technique for intercourse in any position. You can also add to your repertoire by mixing in a variety of speeds, going from slow to fast and then to slow again, for example. Think of your sex life as an ongoing experiment in looking for new and perhaps more fun ways to do things that may have become routine or that you seem to do by just going through the motions without any real feeling. When I'm inside Vera's vagina, I really enjoy pressing my pelvis against her bottom and just lingering there, feeling the sensation spread from my genitals to my entire body.

It is fun to talk to your partner during intercourse—not about business or other mundane topics, of course. Talk about the fun and pleasure you're experiencing, or talk "nasty," or verbalize a fantasy if that turns you on. Many people take and have intercourse very seriously. They do it in the dark, in the missionary position, with neither person saying anything and the woman hoping the guy will ejaculate quickly so they can be finished. If this sounds like you, there is a whole new world of wonderful pleasure out there for you to experience. Make love with the lights on. Get a book on sexual positions and try a bunch of different ones to find a few new favorites. Practice talking with your partner. At first this may seem challenging because we are so conditioned not to talk during sex. Say a little more each time. It really isn't difficult, and after a short while you will be able to freely communicate with your partner. One way to start is to acknowledge the pleasure you're experiencing, which is always a good idea. When you are having stupendous intercourse, there is never a shortage of wonderful and appreciative comments you can make.

∼ How to Touch an Oversensitive Clitoris ∼

We have met many women who believe that their clitorises are too sensitive to be touched. We described this phenomenon briefly in the last chapter, but because we receive lots of e-mails from people asking about this issue, we want to discuss it in more detail. Many women are afraid either to touch the head of their clitoris themselves or to let anyone else touch them there. Even touching it through the hood can sometimes be too scary or painful for them. However, most, if not all, of the women we have met who say their clitorises are too sensitive to be touched directly, once they've been trained in the proper techniques, have learned to accept, and really enjoy, being touched there.

Certain conditions exist, grouped under the term vulvadynia, that can predispose a woman to feeling pain instead of pleasure in the genital area. The conditions haven't been thoroughly studied, and there seems to be controversy over whether they are physical or psychological in nature. It is probably a combination of both. The condition affects only a very small percentage of the population. We have never met a woman who had any kind of actual physical problem with her clitoris. Possible conditions along these lines may exist in the medical literature, but among the many hundreds of clients we have had, none have suffered any clitoral ailments. We have met a few women who were enduring an outbreak of herpes or who claimed to have some form of vulvadynia, but these conditions affect the inner or outer labia or the perineum, never the clitoris. Still, if a woman is unsure about the health of her clitoris, it would be a good idea for her to check with her gynecologist before proceeding with her EMO studies.

According to Natalie Angier, author of *Woman: An Intimate Geography,* the head of the clitoris has approximately eight thousand nerve endings. Stimulating these nerve endings produces a sensation of pressure that an individual can interpret in many different ways. Many women relate this sensation to pleasure and enjoy being stimulated there. Because of the way a woman's body is wired this is the best place to touch her to bring her to orgasm. However, if a woman believes that stimulating the clitoral nerve endings will feel painful or unpleasant, then she won't give herself permission to surrender to the touch and therefore will not feel pleasure but may instead feel pain or discomfort.

Some people believe that sex and pleasure should be comfortable. This is another idea that can cause some problems. Pleasure is way past comfort on the scale of experiences, and if one settles for comfort, one may be unable to open up to more extreme sensations. Comfort means doing things and being in places that are familiar and secure. An intense orgasm can be eye-opening, expansive, thrilling—and also frightening. Because of this fear factor some people would prefer to continue experiencing only what they are familiar with and avoid the risk of what could be a daunting scenario. This can be true no matter what stage of pleasure training a person might be in—from not wanting to be touched at all on the clitoris, to being scared to go to that next, intense level involving a full-body orgasmic response.

Some women's comfort zone is quite shallow and they would prefer not to experience the intense sensations caused by directly touching their clitoris. If a person really does not want to experience more pleasure (a statement that seems almost oxymoronic), then there is nothing that can be done to convince them otherwise. However, most women we've encountered who've been afraid to have their clitorises stimulated would like to learn how to overcome this fear and proceed to much greater pleasure. If a person has deep psychological problems or a history of intensely negative sexual experiences, we refer them to therapy. In most cases the problems are not that deep, and with the proper training a person can learn to be touched in all kinds of ways. The approach must be slow and deliberate to ensure that they will open up instead of closing down and getting defensive.

In almost any sensual encounter with a woman it works best if one doesn't start by going directly for the clitoris or even for the genitals, which we call "crotch diving." This is most important when dealing with someone who is afraid to be touched directly on the clitoris. The best approach is a slow and teasing one. Start by talking and asking questions. Find out what turns her on, and play with those ideas. Touch her in her other erogenous zones—the farther away from the genitals the better—and progressively advance toward the genitals. Have the clitoris be your final destination. Start by kissing her on her lips or neck or even touching her arms or feet with your hands. Enjoy the touch; do it so that it feels good to your hands or lips. Following this approach is the best way to ensure that it feels good to her as well.

Sometimes it can be fun to help her out of her clothes. You may want to get naked, too. Or she can take her own clothes off. You can do the same or even remain clothed. When you're fully clothed and your partner is naked it sometimes can be easier for your partner to surrender to the experience because she does not have to feel any anxiety about reciprocating. At other times, of course, it is lots of fun to be naked together or to be almost naked (wearing a little clothing can often be more erotic than being completely naked). If she is lying down, you can get in a good position to touch her in different areas, starting at her head or feet, for example, and moving to her nipples and breast area.

The idea is to give pleasure by enjoying your touching. You can use your fingertips, hands, wrists, arms, legs, hair, or any other part of the body that feels good to you and that your partner feels okay with. If she does not appreciate being touched with your feet or certain other body parts, then of course don't do that. This is why it is good to know your partner's likes and dislikes and to learn about them as soon as you can.

Once you work your way to her genitals, get into a position in which you feel comfortable (comfort is required here). We recommend a sitting position, which is excellent for being able to talk and touch easily and to see what you are doing. For an illustration of a good position, see Figure 7.1 on page 170.

It is also a good idea to inform your partner about what you are going to do next. If you are going to play with her pubic hair or touch her inner lips, tell her so in advance. Surprise is not a good tactic when you are aiming to gain the trust and confidence of your partner. The more she can feel safe with you in these circumstances, the more willing she will be to allow you to play with her nervous system. Touch around her genitals in any playful and fun way that you can think of. Use your fingers, the back of your hand, the hair on your arm—whatever feels good to you. Continue to avoid touching her clitoris. Use a light and loving caress to touch her pubic hair, inner lips, perineum, and all over her genitals except the clitoris. Tease her by getting close to the clitoris and then backing off.

Now get some lubricant and spread it around her perineum and inner lips, but still resist touching her clitoris. Have fun as you titillate all those genital nerve endings while you spread the lubricant. Find out where she likes to be stimulated. Use a light touch with one finger at a time. Remember to stroke for your own pleasure. You can ask her questions that she can answer with a yes or no, such as: "Would you like more pressure?" "Would you like less pressure?" "Would you like to be touched more to the left?" "Would you like it more to the right?" Check out different areas on her genitals. Stay in one spot or area as long as it is fun for everyone. As long as you are touching for your own pleasure, you can't go wrong.

You can again approach her clitoris along her inner labia and then back off. Tease her so that she will want to be touched. Do this as long as it is fun. Now take some extra lubricant and barely touch the hood of her clitoris with it. See if she pulls back or wants more. If she wants more, you can pull back the hood of the clitoris with your other hand and lightly place some lubricant directly on the clitoral head. Do not allow your finger to touch the clitoris, only the lubricant. To accomplish this we recommend using a good-sized dab of petroleum jelly rather than a thinner, water-based lubricant. Remember to tell her what you are about to do before you do it. As long as she doesn't pull back, you can actually rub the clitoris with the lubricant for a few strokes, still without touching it directly with your fingertip.

Keep your attention on your partner to make sure she isn't going to pull away from you, either emotionally or physically. As long as she is coming toward you, it is okay to proceed and allow a little contact between your finger and the head of the clitoris. If you sense she has had enough or will pull away, it is okay to stop the procedure and thank her for the opportunity. As long as you stop before she does, she will want to do it again soon. The next time, she will let you go a little further. As long as she wants more, you can slowly increase the pressure a little bit at a time. Use a light stroke that just barely touches her clitoris. Many women who come to us with this problem allow us to continue the experience once they realize that they feel no ill effects and that we will stop on a dime if necessary. There is no rush to use regular or moderate pressure, as some women prefer a lighter pressure anyway.

We have found that most women who originally thought their clitoris was too sensitive to be touched learn to appreciate manual contact and actually feel grateful for the experience. They discover their ability to function and be pleasured normally, and they go on to achieve great orgasmic pleasure via direct clitoral stimulation.

~

Doing the exercises in this book and practicing the techniques with a partner can help both men and women become better lovers. Know that it will take time to hone some of the skills to a level where you feel confident about your abilities. Enjoy practicing, and give your partner some leeway in his or her performance. Grant your partner wins when appropriate and positive direction when suitable. Remember that the most important aspect of a great sex life is to have fun in every moment, even when you are learning new skills.

✧ EXERCISE 8A ✧
Orgasm on the First Stroke

Both the clitoris and the head of the penis contain thousands of nerve endings, which can be stimulated to achieve orgasm on the first stroke. We have been conditioned to believe that it takes time to reach orgasm. Most people do this by tensing up until the release, which actually causes them to miss out on most of the sensation that happens along the way. As we explained in Chapter 5, orgasm is not equal to ejaculation or to the "crotch sneeze" at the end, but rather can start from the first moment when you place your attention on your genitals and feel the pleasure and sensation emanating from all those spectacular nerve endings.

In this exercise the woman agrees to receive the attention and her partner agrees to give the attention. The woman lies down, and her partner sits perpendicular to her in a comfortable position where he can easily see and touch her genitals. Instead of stroking her multiple times he is going to touch her clitoris only once. The woman must be as relaxed as possible; this means her partner must remind her to relax.

Start by teasing her around the clitoris for as long as doing so is fun for you. Play with her pubic hair, gently stroking it with either your fingers or the back of your hand or even your wrist. Make the clitoris the focal point. This means you focus your attention on it, even though you touch her *everywhere else but* the clitoris. Touch her inner lips, separate them, apply pressure above her clitoris to pull back the hood (the skin covering the clitoris), and expose the clitoris to the air. Gently apply her favorite lubricant to the areas around her clitoris, reminding her that you will touch the clitoris itself when you are ready. Approach the clitoris from all sides and then retreat. Hopefully your actions will drive her wild and she will already be experiencing orgasmic pleasure with just the thought of her clitoris being touched. Finally, when you feel she totally wants your finger, use your lubricated index finger to give her a single stroke on the exposed clitoris. Report all the sensation you feel.

This completes the exercise. Apply some firm pressure around her clitoris, but not on it, and towel her off.

There are other variations on this theme. You can do two or three strokes and stop. You can do a single stroke, then stop, then do another round of teasing, and then do another stroke. A woman can do this exercise to her man, too. Make the focal point the apex, or underside, of his penis, right below the corona (see Figure 5.4 on page 128). Teasing with words and with light strokes around the clitoris (or the apex of the penis) is a wonderful technique to use at the beginning of practically every orgasmic experience.

✦ EXERCISE 8B ✦
Extending the Orgasm

For a superior orgasm we like to divide the roles of the two participants. One person is the giver of the orgasm and the other person is the receiver. The receiver only has to lie down, relax as much as possible, and put their attention on their pleasure. The giver of the orgasm must take control of the receiver's sexual energy or level of tumescence. The giver does this by focusing their attention on the other person and also by noticing what they are feeling in their own body.

Remember, once you start rubbing on someone else's clitoris or penis, you must stroke it for your own pleasure; that is, touch it because doing so feels wonderful to you. Keep repeating the exact same stroke over and over as long as the sensation continues to feel wonderful and you are enjoying doing it. At some point either the stroking will feel slightly less wonderful or you will have the thought that the next stroke or so won't be as fantastic. This is the time to peak your partner, which means to deliberately bring them down a little. Do this by either stopping, taking a break, or changing the stroke. If you change the stroke before your partner is quite ready for you to, you will take him or her down a little. Then, when you continue with a new stroke, your partner's level of sensation will again increase quickly. If you take a break by removing your hands altogether, the length of the break should depend on how soon you feel like starting to stroke again. When you restart, you can use the same stroke or a different one. Peaking your partner—deliberately bringing them down right before they were going to come down on their own—keeps you in control of your partner's orgasm.

In order to keep the orgasm going you must be sure that your partner is relaxed rather than tensing up. Tensing up will cause your partner to ejaculate (if he's a man) or to experience a "don't touch me anymore" release (if she's a woman). You can get your partner to relax just by asking him or her to relax more. His or her body will respond automatically. Before starting, you can communicate to your partner that at some point in the exercise you will ask him or her to relax. Tell your partner that he or she needn't do anything to respond to your request, only to hear it, in which case his or her body will respond automatically. Your partner can also use the "pushing out" exercise (Exercise 6C) to help him or her relax, even if he's a man.

Before you start, we recommend that you agree upon a time limit for your partner's orgasm. Then, when the time is up, you can decide if you both want to continue. It is also okay to end before the time limit expires.

❦ *Chapter Highlights*

◆ Your feelings will not lie to you, and if you can trust them and express them to your partner in a respectful and kind way, you will raise your sexual expertise to a higher level.

◆ One must learn one's craft in order to be the best lover that anyone would want to have.

◆ The only way your partner can reap the most fun from being your pleasure victim is if you are thoroughly enjoying producing pleasure with him or her.

◆ It can be useful to stay one step ahead of your pleasure victim by anticipating when they may resist and throwing them a curveball when they are likely expecting a fastball down the center of the plate.

◆ When first learning to give your partner an EMO, it may be a good idea to do it only for short periods of time in order to build up your ability to stay attentive and focused for longer.

◆ As long as your intentions and the outcome are at odds, you will remain out of control of the experience.

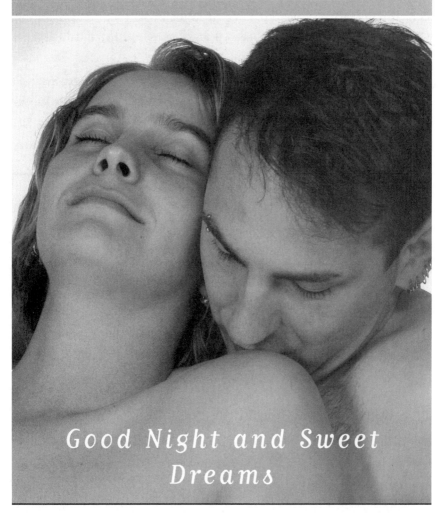

CHAPTER 9

*Good Night and Sweet
Dreams*

*L*ife is not a fairy tale and not everybody is going to live
*happily ever after. However, we believe that if you
choose the right person to live your life with, and if you*
learn your craft as a man to become a magnificent lover and as a woman to
choose pleasure over conditioning, your chances for happiness will definitely
increase.

One does not have to be in a relationship to have a wonderful and full life.
There are other games to play besides the woman/man game, but few are as

all-consuming. If you have come this far in the book, you, like us, probably believe that the best life a person can live is one that is shared with another person—a person whom you love and who loves you.

We hope this book has provided some beneficial information that will make your life more fun. We believe that learning and practicing the lessons we've included here can help you create a more intimate relationship. The fact that you were willing to purchase this book and then to read it all the way through is a sign that you are on your way to a more pleasurable and fulfilling life.

We will not be there to hold your hand through every tricky situation that comes up, but we offer our e-mail address in case you have any problems that you are unable to handle on your own or with the input of your friends: verasteve@aol.com. You can also visit our website at extendedmassiveorgasm.com. Consider finding other couples who are in a situation similar to yours so you have someone to talk to when you encounter roadblocks. It is always easier to solve someone else's problems than it is one's own, and having friends to discuss things with can alleviate some of the frustrations that can arise when a couple is isolated. Plus, sometimes helping other folks with their problems can show you your own challenges in a new light, spawning ideas that can be beneficial to you. We like to say that the course is for the teacher, and we find that we usually learn something helpful for our own lives each time we help someone else. In other words, what goes around comes around, or you reap what you sow.

Women, it is especially important for you to seek out the company of other women who are inclined to support your relationship, as opposed to hanging out with women who like to blame men for all their problems. All too often we have seen women in restaurants and other public places discussing how awful and stupid the men in their lives are. You can also use your women friends to help you train your man; sometimes it indeed takes a village. For example, if you do not trust your fashion sense but you want to help your man dress better, bring along a girlfriend to help you select clothes for him. Whereas he may be able to resist your individual efforts, the combined energies of you and another woman will prove that much more persuasive.

You can also be a friend to other women. If a woman says and does things that are offensive, either to a man or to another woman, chances are she knows, on some level at least, what she is doing and the effect of what she did or said, because most women have more social aptitude than men. That is why, when you witness a woman doing or saying something harmful, it would be doing her a favor to call her on it and to ask her some serious questions about her intentions. Of course, before judging a person solely on the basis of gender, it is always a good idea to view him or her as an individual and to give them as much benefit of the doubt as you can. We are only pointing out these differences to give you a heads-up about what might be occurring so you can act accordingly.

A man will never leave a woman who is appreciative of him and who makes him feel like a hero in bed. Because men crave success and will even choose it over pleasure, if you cause your man to win with you in bed, you will have a happy man. To do this you have to learn how to receive intense pleasure. You cannot just tell him that he is great in bed when you are having some poor excuse for an orgasm. You can only fake pleasure for so long before he catches on. Faking it is self-defeating anyhow. No, to create a hero in bed you must learn to get off well, give up your anger, and become an extremely fun human being.

Not every topic we've discussed in this book will apply equally to everyone. We really have covered the full range of relationship issues—from finding a partner, to dating, to creating great sensual pleasure, to moving in together, to marrying, and beyond. Still, we think the information offered in each chapter and about each subject can be helpful to you even if your relationship is in a different stage from what's being discussed. In addition, people and relationships come in many variations, though most readers will see parts of themselves in at least some of the descriptions.

We wrote this book in part because we wanted to share aspects of our lives and some of the important lessons we have learned. Some of these lessons we learned the hard way: We each were married twice before finding each other. A lot of our experience came from our years of living communally, taking courses, and teaching classes at an experimental school in Northern California.

There, we studied orgasm as well as alternative lifestyles. As a group we were kind of like guinea pigs. Some of our research involved how men and women could relate better to one another—that is, in a more open and communicative way. People had affairs, just like they do in normal society, but everything was aboveboard and there were few or no secrets. People still got jealous, but because everyone was willing to take responsibility for their actions and their lives, it was a lot less dramatic than it would have been if people had been having secret affairs that were discovered by chance.

A lot of the information in this book also comes from what we've learned while helping our students. We have been facilitating people's creation of more enjoyable relationships and better sex lives for over twenty years, thirteen of those outside of the experimental school. Every time someone has a question, it can open up a new adventure for us as well as for them as we decide what to expose to them about our lives that could possibly help them in theirs.

We feel fortunate to have met one another when we did and under the circumstances that we did. We do not believe we would have become a couple if we had met anywhere other than where and when we did. Vera was married and thirteen years my senior, and I was single and had no money. Yet we liked each other's inner being from the beginning, so we developed a love affair that continues to grow after more than twenty-two years of marriage. In part this is because when we got together we had friends whom we could share with and learn from. Then, because we continued to assist others who asked for our help, we were able to take our friendship and love to an even higher level.

This book is about more than being a goddess or a hero in bed. Reading it will give you a greater understanding of what it takes to build a wonderful and intimate relationship. The game of love between a woman and a man involves your whole being. To play it requires all of your attention at certain times, and certainly some of your attention all of the time. The reward is a life that is shared with another human being, a partnership that permits you to be fully yourself, and to totally reveal that self to a witness and a friend. It is a game in which two different people come to know one another better all the time, while learning and growing from the experience. It is the union of aliens into a team that can do things that neither member could do on his or her own. It creates a whole that is greater than the sum of its parts. The obstacles and possible pitfalls are many, but with desire and the right attitude, the willingness to make use of one's friends, and any other resources that can be of assistance, the players can create heaven on earth. Those who choose this path are consciously choosing pleasure. They are choosing to go to bed.

I'm thrilled!
You are not me.
Your generosity is contagious
You are smooth and silky
Your beauty is outrageous.
I'm hairy and bony,
Watch out for those knees and elbows.
You like it hot!
I prefer things cool.
I bend
You follow the rule.
You like closets closed,
So I leave them open.
I love women!
As you love men.
You make people feel at ease.
I was born to tease.
You love to buy,
I'd rather sell.
I see a pattern forming.
You see random delight!

You say thank you and please,
I resist to appease.
You stack everything neat,
I throw things in a heap.
You choose the train
I prefer the plane.
You eat butter and cheese,
Why not drink green teas?
You can be so stubborn,
As I bend like an oak.
You've got curves
I've got lines.
We fit perfectly
Even our signs.
Difference adds life.
If we were the same,
There would be no wonder,
There would be no game.
Let's go to bed!

Bibliography

Angier, Natalie. *Woman: An Intimate Geography*. New York: Houghton Mifflin, 1999.

Baranco, Vic. *I Dogma: Vol. 1*. Lafayette, CA: More University Press, 1986.

Bodansky, Vera and Steve. *Extended Massive Orgasm*. Alameda, CA: Hunter House, 2000.

Bodansky, Vera and Steve. *The Illustrated Guide to Extended Massive Orgasm*. Alameda, CA: Hunter House, 2002.

Deyo, Yaacov and Sue. *Speed Dating: The Smarter, Faster Way to Lasting Love*. New York: Harper Resource, 2002.

Gilman, Susan Jane. *Kiss My Tiara: How to Rule the World as a SmartMouth Goddess*. New York: Warner Books, 2001.

Greene, Robert. *The Art of Seduction*. New York: Viking Penguin Putnam, 2001.

Fisher, Helen. *The Sex Contract: The Evolution of Human Behavior*. New York: William Morrow, 1982.

Heinlein, Robert A. *Time Enough for Love*. Berkeley, CA: G.P. Putnam Sons, 1973.

Morinis, Alan. *Climbing Jacob's Ladder: One Man's Rediscovery of a Jewish Spiritual Trait*. New York: Broadway Books, 2002.

Schlain, Leonard. *The Alphabet Versus the Goddess: The Conflict Between Word and Image*. New York: Penguin Putnam, 1998.

Sterling, Justin. *What Really Works with Men.* New York: Warner Books, 1992.

Tavris, Carol. *The Mismeasure of Women: Why Women Are Not the Better Sex, the Inferior Sex, or the Opposite Sex.* New York: Touchstone, 1993.

Thomashauer, Regena. *Mama Gena's School of Womanly Arts: Using the Power of Pleasure to Have Your Way with the World.* New York: Simon and Schuster, 2002.

Thomashauer, Regena. *Mama Gena's Owner's and Operator's Guide to Men.* New York: Simon and Schuster, 2003.

Zuk, Marlene. *Sexual Selections: What We Can and Can't Learn about Sex from Animals.* Berkeley: University of California Press, 2002.

Index

A

affairs, 83–86

African Queen, 147–148

alcohol, and the sensual experience, 109–110

Alphabet Versus the Goddess, The (Schlain), 4

anger, 99–104, 105, 141

Angier, Natalie, 206

appearance, importance of, 15–17

appetite, components of, 46–48

arguments, 66–72

arousal, 126–127

Art of Seduction, The (Greene), 48

attractiveness, 15–17, 46, 75

B

babies, 82

Baranco, Vic, 79, 95, 100, 165, 201

Beauty and the Beast, 147–148

bed: as metaphor, 1, 9, 115; quality of, 1, 9

blind-spot castration, 177–179

C

children, 82

Climbing Jacob's Ladder (Morinis), 61, 103

clitoris, 141; guide for men, 167–173; hood, 168–170, 172; how to stroke, 171–172; importance of, 88–90, 95; oversensitivity, 205–209; paying attention to, 142–144; quadrants of, 170–171

comfort zone, 206–207

communication, 35–55; hurt, admitting to, 41–42; interpreting womanese, 39–41; lack of, 44–46; paying attention, 36–37; what not to say, 42–44; what to say, 37–39

compliments, importance of paying, 37

confidence, 24–28, 193–194

conflicts, 66–72

control, 191–193

counseling, 85

courtship, 11–12

cunnilingus, 175–177

curiosity, 197–199

D

dating. *See* partners

Deyo, Sue, 29

Deyo, Yaacov, 29

dress, importance of, 15–17

drugs and the sensual experience, 109–110

E

ejaculation, 128–129

EMO (extended massive orgasm), 130, 179; for men, 173–174

emotions, expressing, 60–61

engorgement, loss of, 164–165

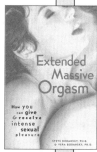
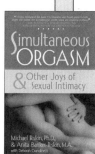

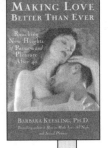

FEMALE EJACULATION & THE G-SPOT

by Deborah Sundahl ... Forewords by Annie Sprinkle and Alice Ladas

Discover the G-spot's hidden sensations of intense pleasure ...
The G-spot is a woman's prostate gland. When stimulated, it swells
with blood and emits ejaculate fluid, usually during orgasm.
All women have a G-spot, and all women can ejaculate.
Author Deborah Sundahl has led seminars on female ejacu-
lation for 15 years, and this book is based on her research.
Contents include:

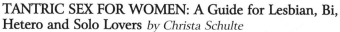

   ** techniques and positions that help a woman ejaculate

   ** how men can help their female partners to ejaculate

Massage techniques developed by body-work specialists
and Tantric healers are included along with exercises to help
release emotional pain.

240 pages ... 13 illus. ... Paperback $15.95

TANTRIC SEX FOR WOMEN: A Guide for Lesbian, Bi, Hetero and Solo Lovers *by Christa Schulte*

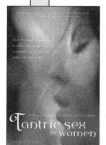

Every woman can enhance her sexual experiences through
the use of Tantra. Christa Schulte, a longtime practitioner,
introduces women to *Tara-Tantra,* a woman-centered
approach that she has developed and taught for many years.

   Over 50 exercises are included ... for solo-lovers, love
games for two, rituals, meditations, and massage techniques, all designed to enable women to fulfill their sexual
and sensual potential, enrich their relationships, and enjoy
the small ecstasies of everyday life. The book will also help
men who want to understand women's sexuality more
deeply and become more fulfilling partners.

288 pages ... 2 illus. ... 14 b/w photos ... Paperback $15.95

WOMEN'S SEXUAL PASSAGES: Finding Pleasure and Intimacy at Every Stage of Life *by Elizabeth Davis*

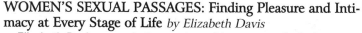

Elisabeth Davis unravels the mystery of how women's desire
changes in the course of her lifetime under the influence of biologi-
cal rhythms, menstruation, pregnancy, birth, child rearing, cultural
attitudes, menopause, and aging. She helps women understand the
effects of stress, relationship upheaval, and sexual abuse, and new
chapters address sex in the later years and how hormonal changes
at menopause can bring greater insight and assertiveness.

288 pages ... 1 illus ... Paperback $15.95

THE HOT GUIDE TO SAFER SEX *by Yvonne Fulbright, M.S.Ed.*

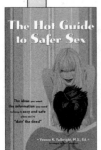

Safer sex and erotic romps have always been considered mutually exclusive. Enter Yvonne Fulbright, a sexuality instructor and bonafide "sexpert." She tackles the subject in a hip, entertaining tone, packs the book with information and research findings, and introduces readers to techniques that lower their risk of getting an STD while improving the overall quality of their sexual experiences.

Chapters include: "Sacred Spots and Erogenous Zones," "You Always Can in Fantasyland," "Horny & High: What Drugs Really Do to Your Sex Life," "So You Want Something to Play With," and "Making a Multi-Orgasmic Man."

352 pages ... Paperback $14.95

SENSUAL SEX: Awakening Your Senses and Deepening the Passion in Your Relationship *by Beverly Engel, MFCC*

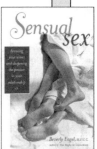

Life is a sensual experience that we can smell, taste, touch—and enjoy. *Sensual Sex* brings that dimension to lovemaking. The one-of-a-kind "Reawakening Your Senses" program engages couples in a whole new level of physical exploration, "Deeper Love" offers an introduction to Tantric sex and sexual ecstasy, and "The Four Seasons of Sensuous Passion" discusses the stages of intimate relationships and sensual exercises that can strengthen each phase. Sensitively written and beautifully designed, this is a book to share, enjoy, and keep for a long time.

256 pages ... 18 illus. ... Paperback $14.95

SEX TIPS & TALES FROM WOMEN WHO DARE: Exploring the Exotic Erotic. *Edited by Jo-Anne Baker. Contributors include Deborah Sundahl, Susie Bright, Annie Sprinkle, Joani Blank, Linda Montano, Jwala, Veronica Vera, Carol Queen, Kat Sunlove, Candida Royalle, Nan Kinney, and Nina Hartley.*

A remarkable collection of writings by women at the forefront of the sexual revolution — from journalists and entrepreneurs to porn stars and transsexuals — who share intimate secrets on sex, self-love, and satisfaction. Their writings provide a stimulating perspective on sexuality as a life-long adventure.

"Dynamic and delicious..."
— Eve Ensler, author of *The Vagina Monologues*

256 pages. ... 30 b/w photos ... Paperback $13.95

Order online at www.hunterhouse.com ... all prices subject to change

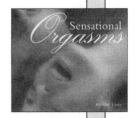
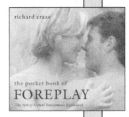
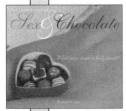
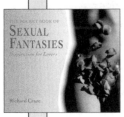

ORDER FORM

10% DISCOUNT on orders of $50 or more —
20% DISCOUNT on orders of $150 or more —
30% DISCOUNT on orders of $500 or more —
On cost of books for fully prepaid orders

NAME

ADDRESS

CITY/STATE   ZIP/POSTCODE

PHONE   COUNTRY (outside of U.S.)

TITLE	*QTY*	*PRICE*	*TOTAL*
To Bed or Not to Bed (paper)		@ $ 14.95	
Extended Massive Orgasm (paper)		@ $ 14.95	

Prices subject to change without notice

Please list other titles below:

		@ $	
		@ $	
		@ $	
		@ $	
		@ $	
		@ $	
		@ $	

Check here to receive our book catalog ☐   *FREE*

Shipping Costs		
By Priority Mail: first book $4.50, each additional book $1.00	TOTAL	
	Less discount @_____%	(_____)
By UPS and to Canada: first book $5.50, each additional book $1.50	TOTAL COST OF BOOKS	_____
	Calif. residents add sales tax	_____
For rush orders and other countries call us at (510) 865-5282	Shipping & handling	_____
	TOTAL ENCLOSED	======
	Please pay in U.S. funds only	

☐ Check   ☐ Visa   ☐ MasterCard   ☐ Discover

Card #_____ Exp. date_____

Signature_____

Complete and mail to:
Hunter House Inc., Publishers
PO Box 2914, Alameda CA 94501-0914
Website: www.hunterhouse.com
Orders: (800) 266-5592 or email: ordering@hunterhouse.com
Phone (510) 865-5282   Fax (510) 865-4295

TBN 12/2005